SELF-INQUIRY

16 June 2011

For Barbara,
With great love.

Swamiji

Also by Swami Shankarananda

Happy for No Good Reason
Consciousness Is Everything
Carrot in My Ear

Available from Shaktipat Press

SELF-INQUIRY

USING YOUR AWARENESS TO UNBLOCK YOUR LIFE

SWAMI SHANKARANANDA

SHAKTIPAT
PRESS

Published by Shaktipat Press, 2008
27 Tower Road, Mt Eliza
Victoria 3930
Australia
Telephone: +61 3 9775 2568 Fax: +61 3 9775 2591
email: askus@shivayoga.org
www.shivayoga.org

The National Library of Australia
Cataloguing-in-Publication data:

Shankarananda, Swami.
Self-inquiry: using your awareness to unblock your life/author, Swami Shankarananda.

ISBN 978-0-9750995-3-7

Includes index.
Bibliography.

Meditation. Yoga. Spirituality. Self-actualization (Psychology).
Self (Philosophy). Self-realization.

294.543

Design: Kali Nolle
Back cover photo: Peter Cassamento
Printed in Australia by BPA Print Group

For Devi Ma.
When I sought to create a method of Self-inquiry,
you were sent to me.
You were there at the beginning, the middle and the end.
You are the muse and deity of this work.

ACKNOWLEDGMENTS

This book is the result of years of spiritual work and experimentation in which many people took part. First, I want to acknowledge my great Guru, Swami Muktananda, in whose presence my understanding of Self-inquiry was inspired. Later, when I asked the question, he said 'yes'.

I bow to the great sages, especially Ramana Maharshi, who blazed the way.

Next, I want to acknowledge Devi Ma, to whom I dedicate this book. She has worked with the process over many years, helping me shape it with her unmatched intuition.

I must acknowledge my editor, Jacqueline Bos, who worked with me on the text, selflessly giving up her spare time. She held every idea and thought in her mind and always knew when one of my additions was valuable or repetitive. I couldn't have done it without you Jackie.

Let me acknowledge my dear Professor Patrick Mahaffey, Chair of Mythological Studies Program at Pacifica Graduate Institute, Santa Barbara, California, for his sensitive and insightful foreword.

As always, I am indebted to Kali Nolle for the print design of the book and the cover. She turns my books into objects of beauty.

Thank you to Swami Dayananda for creating the index and reading and rereading the text, offering advice on content and structure. Kaymolly Morrelle also read through the text many times and did much valuable copyediting. Thanks also to Dr Jo Hughson for checking the Sanskrit and for general assistance.

And I want to thank Daniel Vuillermin for producing the CD that goes with the book, and Jim Walter who assisted with the mixing.

Thank you to Dr Gary Witus for his suggestions and to Dylan Frusher, Mary-Anne MacCallum and Leigh Saward who helped in various ways. And also to Sandy Kouroupidis who organised the printing, and to Dr Isobel Crombie who transcribed the lectures.

I also must acknowledge Mother Girija, Danny Greenberg and the members of the original Ann Arbor inquiry groups. Also, Amma, who said 'no'.

Finally, I salute all the Shiva Yogis and inquiry practitioners who have worked with me for the past 20 years, giving their heart and soul to the process of Self-discovery. It is because of their dedication to the truth that this method of Self-inquiry is honed and powerful.

ACKNOWLEDGMENTS

*They in whom the spirit of inquiry is ever awake illumine the world,
enlighten all who come in contact with them, dispel the ghosts created by an
ignorant mind ... In the light of inquiry there is realisation of the eternal
and unchanging reality ... [One who practises inquiry] is free from delusion
and attachment ... he lives and functions in this world and reaches the
blissful state of total freedom.*
Yoga Vashishta

*... though truth and falsehood be
Near twins, yet truth a little elder is;
Be busy to seek her, believe me this,
... To stand inquiring right, is not to stray;
To sleep, or run wrong, is. On a huge hill,
Cragged and steep, Truth stands, and he that will
Reach her, about must and about must go,
And what the hill's suddenness resists, win so ...*
John Donne

*Good judgment comes from experience,
and a lot of that comes from bad judgment.*
Will Rogers

*Seek what is immediate and intimate
rather than what is distant and unknown.*
Sri Ramana Maharshi

CONTENTS

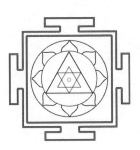

FOREWORD

THE GREAT WISDOM traditions teach methods for spiritual awakening. These paths help individuals attain self-knowledge through the careful observation of their life experiences. The pre-eminent method for expanding awareness in Indian spirituality is called Self-inquiry (*atma vichara*) and is associated with the path of discriminating knowledge or wisdom (*jnana* yoga). This process originated in the ancient literature of the *Upanishads* and it has been kept alive and revitalised by Vedantic sages such as Sri Shankaracharya and 20th-century teachers like Sri Ramana Maharshi and Sri Nisargadatta Maharaj. Fortunately for us, Swami Shankarananda continues this practice to the present day in a form that is both traditional and remarkably innovative. This book conveys the essence of his method of Self-inquiry in a manner that exemplifies his clear and engaging teaching style.

The aim of Self-inquiry is to discover and realise the Self. Traditionally it is a path of negation or *via negativa*. A person discovers their innermost being by disidentifying with what one is not: the body, thoughts, feelings and other characteristics that typically constitute identity such as gender, age and occupation. This is the approach of Ramana Maharshi, the sage who is most frequently associated with Self-inquiry. Swami Shankarananda provides an illuminating account of this method and demonstrates how we may experience its efficacy in our own lives. However, he observes that Ramana's method is uncompromising. It aims at silencing the mind so that one may experience the pristine awareness of the Self. Shankarananda endeavours to bring Self-inquiry down to earth: he gives it a body, a mind and a voice. While spirituality may be the most important aspect of life, he honours the fact that our bodies, work and relationships also deserve our attention. In actuality, each of these areas of life is intimately related to our spirituality. All of them express our life force, and the purpose of Self-inquiry is to remove the blocks that obstruct its flow.

Swamiji often says that a sage teaches the path that he himself has walked. This is certainly true in his case. His example inspires us to realise our own greatness. His form of Self-inquiry emerged 35 years ago in Ganeshpuri, India, while he was doing *sadhana*, spiritual practice, in the presence of his Guru, Swami Muktananda. In the late '80s, he began to teach a guided meditation technique based on the Self-inquiry he had first discovered in India. By the '90s, he began to offer Self-inquiry groups at his ashram in Australia and he named his method the *Shiva Process*. This approach, both in its personal inquiry and group-inquiry forms, is central to his teaching and is an integral part of the practices done at his ashram. He lives there among his students and devotees, empowering them to courageously put forth their best efforts to be better human beings.

I recently spent a month in residence at Swamiji's ashram while on sabbatical from my academic position. My intention was to deepen my understanding of Kashmir Shaivism, the philosophy that deeply informs his teachings on meditation and yoga. My experience there greatly exceeded my expectations. Not only did I gain a better understanding of the core teachings of Shaivite yoga, I also learned how to practise these ideas in the context of a community of yogis who exhibited an astonishing degree of emotional maturity. Ashram residents and householders alike demonstrated their ability to 'walk the talk' in a down-to-earth and natural manner. And they had a sense of humour, too! What accounted for this? The answer was clear. It was their commitment to practising Self-inquiry. This moment-to-moment way of paying attention to experience grounded other practices like meditation and chanting, and provided a means for integrating their effects into the fabric of work, relationships and leisure activities.

The Shiva Process is a practical application of Kashmir Shaivism's teachings about *matrika*; the power of language. Shaivism says that we create our reality by means of inner language and the language we use in everyday life. Our feelings often conceal negative thoughts and our negative thoughts in turn generate emotions such as anger and fear. If feelings are repressed or disavowed, we become stuck or contracted. If they are brought to awareness, our condition may shift. Shiva Process enables us to transmute our negative feelings and thoughts via the power of awareness.

The Shiva Process method is direct and easy to practise. The practitioner looks inside and asks, 'What is going on here?' while observing the areas of tension within. Using the techniques that Swamiji describes in the book, one recognises and acknowledges the feeling, seeking an *upward shift*. While an upward shift may not occur in every instance, one's awareness is always expanded through this process. We become aware of where we truly stand. Indeed, awareness is what matters most, and the Shiva Process form of Self-inquiry is an excellent tool for learning how to be truly present to what is happening in one's life.

To my knowledge, Swami Shankarananda is the first person to develop a yogic Self-inquiry process for groups. It is a highly innovative way to examine the unconscious. He tells us that 'everyone mirrors everyone' else and the 'space in the centre of the group is a shining mirror of Consciousness' that reflects the unconscious back to participants. Swamiji's favourite metaphor for group process is 'the *yagna*; a Vedic ritual. In this ritual ... Brahmin priests sit around a sacred fire and throw ghee (clarified butter) and other foodstuffs into it' as they chant mantras. 'When the ghee hits the fire, it flares up.' Similarly, Swamiji explains that 'the participants in group-inquiry are like modern-day Brahmins, sitting around the fire of Consciousness'. The group begins in separation, but by following the Shiva Process method, words of 'truth and love' are discovered, which become the ghee that makes 'the fire of awareness blaze brighter'.

Shiva Process Self-inquiry is a form of yoga: the yoga of wisdom. It may also have a significant therapeutic effect on its participants. As a professor at an institute dedicated to the study of depth psychology and the wisdom traditions of different cultures, I am deeply interested in Swamiji's methods of working with the unconscious. He realised early on that inquiry could be a way to join Eastern yoga to Western psychology. Both traditions reduce suffering by helping people deal with afflictive feelings and thoughts that arise from the unconscious. But the differences between the two approaches are also noteworthy.

Swamiji says:

> The ocean is very deep. It has many things hidden within it ... While psychoanalysis tends to plumb the depths of the ocean, in Shiva Process we examine what is thrown up on the beach, moment to moment. In other words, we have faith in the power of Consciousness as it manifests in the present moment. The present moment gives you what you need.

Differences are particularly evident with respect to groups. Group therapy focuses on the people in the group and their stories concerning their troubles. In group-inquiry, the focus is the space at the centre of the group. That space is regarded as Consciousness and represents the relationship or *satsang* of everyone in that moment. As Swamiji puts it, 'It is as though the players build a mandala of feeling together, with the aim of expanding and purifying that feeling. The feeling ... is never one person's problem or one person's fault, but everyone's joint koan'.

Swami Shankarananda's method of Self-inquiry is a path of truth, kindness and peace. It enables us to take responsibility for our lives and our interactions with the world. His message is profoundly life-affirming: 'There is no person, no thought, no object and no emotion that is not Shiva.' The Self is ever-present, blissful and supremely free. Remove the blocks that impede this awareness through inquiry, and connect with the Self. Align yourself with the pulsating Consciousness that exists within your experience and that throbs at the heart of the entire universe.

May all who practise the teachings in this splendid book recognise the Self and abide in peace.

Dr Patrick Mahaffey
Chair, Mythological Studies Program
Pacifica Graduate Institute
Santa Barbara, California
March 2006

INTRODUCTION

AS A SPIRITUAL teacher, I meet many people. I hear sad stories. I've come to the conclusion that the task of being a human being is a difficult one.

When the soul takes on a body, it becomes confused. The physical plane is indeed hard to master. People don't know how to conduct their relationships. They don't know what to say and when to say it. They don't know how to earn a living nor how to save their money. They don't know how to deal with their desires and fears nor how to discipline the energies of their body.

When we are born, we are not given a how-to manual, and the advice we get from our family and culture may be remarkably wrongheaded. Nonetheless, there is an appropriate art of living. The great masters have called this art many things: living in the Tao, Zen, yoga, Tantra, the natural state (*sahaja samadhi*). These names given by different traditions refer to the same thing: a life lived from the centre outward, a life in contact with the Self. Because we are blocked in career and relationship, in the areas of health and wellbeing, we need a method to cut away the misinformation under which we struggle, and get to the truth. Self-inquiry is that method. Self-inquiry gives us a way to deconstruct the false constructions of the mind, and reveal the true Self.

This, then, is a book about Self-inquiry, a subject close to my heart. Self-inquiry is the mother of all spiritual methods and all forms of meditation. It is direct, sleek and effective. It requires no religious belief, nor any dogma to practise it. It is very much in the modern spirit because, like science, it is a quest to discover what *is*.

The need for inquiry becomes critical when we understand that we are broadcasting stations for our feelings. We live life passionately and we always speak and act out of one feeling or another. If we have a negative feeling, like tension, anger, fear or depression, we express that feeling through negative thoughts, negative actions and negative speech. We blame others. Our thoughts, words and deeds express our negativity.

This has a profound impact on our life. If we are broadcasting negativity, other people feel it. We don't get the job we have interviewed for. People move away from us. They avoid our company. Even our pets run away. We may blame circumstances and other people, but the source is in the thoughts and feelings that we are broadcasting through our speech and our actions. As intelligent yogis, we become aware of our negativity, whether by direct instruction or the feedback we are getting from others. Instead of projecting the feeling, we take it inside through Self-inquiry and seek to purify it. We investigate the feeling, release it, relax it and take responsibility for it.

After successful inquiry, our feeling is now positive. We radiate joy, love, peace and confidence, which translate into positive thoughts, positive actions and positive speech. Now we get the job we seek and people want to be around us. Our life is positively transformed by means of Self-inquiry.

The name most linked to Self-inquiry in the history of spirituality is that of the great 20th-century Indian sage, Sri Ramana Maharshi. Ramana said that all methods must necessarily end in inquiry. His reasoning was something like this: you meditate on an image of the deity or the Guru, or you contemplate a spiritual principle, or even look at a *yantra* (sacred diagram). In the end, the question will arise, 'Who is it that is seeing, hearing or experiencing whatever you are meditating on?' And with that question, inquiry begins. The attention moves from the object to the witnessing subject; from the periphery to the centre. Self-inquiry is an inner investigation that moves to the core of reality—ever more inward, more real, more true, more present, more vibrant, more central is its direction and thrust.

I met my Guru, Swami Muktananda (Baba), in Delhi early in 1971. There was a big tent on a sprawling lawn and hundreds of people were attending *satsang*, a spiritual gathering in the company of a great being. In the corner, a young man was sitting in meditation but he was also vibrating, hyperventilating and flopping about like a fish. I'd already heard that Swami Muktananda had a legendary power to awaken the *kundalini* energy, the inner divine power of seekers, and this caused *kriyas*, yogic movements, that were sometimes quite physical or even violent. This was the first one I'd ever seen and I looked at it with a sceptical eye. But it passed the test: I knew it was genuine. Some force other than his own will was moving in that young man. At the same time, an inner knowing arose in me: 'That will not happen to me!'

I was correct in that while I had many spiritual experiences, I never did flop about like a fish. But *shaktipat*, awakening of the *kundalini* energy by the Guru, can manifest in a wide variety of ways. Because of my scepticism, when the energy started coursing through my body forcefully, my first thought was that I might have malaria! Finally I noticed that my 'malaria' was strangely responsive to the evening *Arati* program. I realised I was experiencing an awakening.

In my case, the most significant effect of *shaktipat* was that it drove my mind inward and gave birth to the process of inquiry that has become the Shiva Process. My mind had been exceedingly external; only divine grace could reorient it inwardly.

Feeling frustrated with my efforts to know the Self, I asked Baba for advice. He told me that rather than straining to know the Self conceived of as far away, I should know that the Self is always complete and perfect within me. He said I should contemplate 'I am the Self. I am Shiva'. By Shiva, he was not referring to the Hindu deity of that name, but to universal Consciousness, the substance of the Self. His answer transformed my *sadhana* by 180 degrees. I no longer felt I was striving for some attainment, but rather that the attainment was already present and I had to rediscover it.

According to one yogi, there are two significant obstructions to knowing the Self. One is ignorance of its existence and of the possibility of making contact with it. The other is a tight, cramped state of inner tension. Baba's answer had solved the first, though the latter remained a problem.

On another occasion, I was meditating in the company of my teacher. Feeling on that day the contraction of my being, and frustrated by how far away the goal seemed, I strained to go deeper and have a more profound experience. I felt blocked and discouraged. Suddenly, the understanding arose in me, 'You may not be having the meditation you want, but you can *always* have the meditation you're having'. With it came an intuitive grasp of a completely different spiritual orientation. I would no longer seek something I felt I needed or wanted, but I would now investigate what actually existed. Combining this with Baba's instruction that I should contemplate 'I am the Self', I had the beginnings of a complete method.

Following it, I focus on my inner world, arming myself with his instruction that the Self is already here, already present, though perhaps hidden. I decide to investigate my experience in the very moment. Exploring inwardly, I discover a rich variety of phenomena: movements of energy, subtle feelings and sensations. With my inner eye, I see a number of lights. Most interestingly, I discover blocks and areas of tension in my subtle world. These attract my attention. I can see directly that they affect my wellbeing and my emotional state. The energy of my inner world does not flow properly and harmoniously as long as these tensions remain. I intuit that these blocks, which are more subtle than physical, can eventually manifest as disease.

Acknowledging that these tensions have a profound effect on me as well as on my spiritual state, I feel I've come face to face with my spiritual dilemma as it shows up in the moment. I begin to investigate these perceived blocks. What are they made of? What causes them? I try to get as close to them experientially as I can. I inquire into them and they yield information. My inner voice tells me, 'This is anger. This is fear'. I inquire further. A knowing arises that these tensions are connected to a circumstance that happened today, or a week ago, or even years before. I am starting to unravel the mystery of my inner being.

Sometimes a solution to a block arises in my awareness spontaneously, and when that happens, the block dissolves and I feel a release of tension. My inner being is more harmoniously poised. I leave this meditation in a far more uplifted state than I began it.

I had hit on a method that seemed a universal way of dealing with spiritual obstacles. Where Ramana's inquiry focused only on Self-knowledge, the inquiry I was doing was applicable to all areas of life. I discovered that the problems I encountered with other people, issues of work in the ashram, doubts that arose in my *sadhana*, all showed up within me as tensions and blocks. I could work within myself to release these blocks by finding intuitive means. Having worked on them within, I noticed that obstacles were simultaneously removed from my outer life. My inquiry took wings in the presence of my Guru, and I felt certain that his spiritual energy, his Shakti, brought my inquiry to a boil.

The philosophy of Kashmir Shaivism says that this whole universe is an unfoldment of Consciousness. At the very interior of the universe is divinity, pure light, pure energy and pure love. As Consciousness unfolds externally, things become more gross and material. When we investigate anything, we go in the opposite direction—from the outer to the inner, from the husk to the kernel, from the external to the essence.

In a world of Consciousness, everything is subject to inquiry. When we have a conversation, there are the words that we speak and their meaning, and then deeper down, a more real conversation occurs at the emotional level. The universe is a detective story and becomes, as we move from the periphery to the centre, always more real.

During the years of my *sadhana* at my Guru's feet, I practised and refined this method of inquiry. During those years, I didn't think of it as 'my method of inquiry' but simply as a way to clear myself of whatever toxicity had arisen day to day. Meanwhile, a glimmer of an idea took root in my mind. Perhaps inquiry was a method that could join Eastern yoga to Western psychology.

In 1974, my teacher sent me to found an ashram in Ann Arbor, Michigan. My spiritual practice with him had been intuitive rather than doctrinal, with teachings coming by way of osmosis more than concept. Here, too, when he sent me off to start an ashram, his only instruction was, 'Imitate me'. I did the best I could, and it wasn't bad, but I found that the relationships among the ashramites were difficult.

Baba could yell and shake the earth and frighten everyone into good behaviour, but I couldn't do that. Instead, I saw this as a good opportunity to develop something along the lines I'd been thinking. The ashram could use a psychological group that would be centred in yoga. By the good offices of a notably quirky ashramite named Gilly-Gilly, we were introduced to two therapists who did group work, Danny and Valerie. Valerie would later be known as Ma Devi. I found their work most remarkable.

Everything was in readiness for my experiment, but I needed Baba's approval. In November 1974, Baba visited Columbus, Ohio, and the Ann Arbor staff helped him during his programs, one of which was the Intensive, where participants receive *shaktipat*. I was his chauffeur that week and lived in the back of his house. I approached his chief aide Amma, saying I needed to speak privately to Baba. During the weekend, she set up a meeting for me with Baba, Mother Girija (my then wife and co-director of the Ann Arbor Ashram) and Amma. Before the meeting, I told Amma I wanted to set up an ashram group on Self-inquiry. She said, 'Baba would want you to chant and meditate and do traditional practices'. I said I understood that, but this idea was coming up forcefully inside me. I couldn't let it go without running it by Baba.

At the meeting, I told Baba what I planned in as succinct a way as I could. Amma translated what I said into Hindi for him. Baba answered briefly. Instead of translating what he said, Amma started talking to Baba again. From her tone and body language, I thought she was arguing with his answer. This behaviour was astonishing. Baba seemed displeased and admonished her. Amma turned to me and said, 'Baba says, "Yes, you can do it"'. Baba spoke again. Amma translated: 'Baba said, "Whatever you do, I'm behind you".' I left the room giddy with Baba's support, but troubled by Amma's behaviour.

A day or two later, Baba left Columbus for New York. I drove him to the airport. After a wait, he went through the checkpoint towards the plane. Amma and the other members of his party went through as well. Suddenly, Amma turned around and came back out through the checkpoint to me. She said, 'Baba said "yes", but he meant "no"'.

I was shocked and confused. Still, I was determined to try my experiment. But whether my idea was not yet ripe or because of the impact of Amma's attitude, which haunted me, I gave it up after a few sessions. Was Amma reflecting her own attitude, or did she understand Baba better than I did? Had he said something privately to her? I could not resolve the doubts that had arisen and I put my idea on hold for almost 20 years. Nonetheless, the idea remained in the back of my mind.

Perhaps both Amma and Baba, each in their own way, were right. In my years in Ganeshpuri, Amma was Baba's closest disciple and she often interpreted his teachings to us raw recruits from the West. I had great love and respect for her. I felt she looked out for my interests. In my case, Baba's 'yes' may have meant 'In the fullness of time, I am totally behind you and trust your creative drive. That which you are struggling to find in this "therapy group" is indeed a teaching that lies close to your heart and I completely support your effort to discover it'. Amma's 'no' may have meant 'Whatever the merits of your idea, you must be mindful of the fact that you are at present a disciple and live in the Guru's culture. In a Guru culture, only the Guru himself has licence to initiate major methods. To introduce something so radical would cause problems, especially for you. Later on you might try such experiments, but not now'.

In the late '80s, I began to use a technique of meditation in my Learn to Meditate courses based on the Self-inquiry I had developed during my time in Ganeshpuri. I would ask meditators to get in touch with the feeling in the navel, heart, throat and brow. I asked them if the feeling was pleasant or unpleasant, and to especially notice any unpleasantness or contraction.

Once when a participant had a problem with a strong block in one of the centres, I worked with her there in front of the class. The results were very good: with my help she was able to identify the feeling, the cause of it, and even the solution. During this work and subsequent similar occasions in my meditation classes, I hit on the techniques that later became 'feedback', calling them A- and B-Statements. I gave participants statements that I thought reflected their present condition (A-Statements). Then I asked them to repeat the statements and tell me which ones seemed to fit. Next, I gave them statements that I thought might have an uplifting or pacifying effect (B-Statements) and asked them to repeat those and tell me which were the most effective. This signal success led to other experiments. It became clear I had hit upon a technology that was the fulfilment of the vague ideas that I had, years before, presented to Baba.

I was gratified to discover that I had a way to externalise and teach a process that had been my private means of *sadhana*. Every element of the group-inquiry I discuss later is a stylisation of my internal method that was developed at Baba's feet. I also want to acknowledge the ongoing contribution of Ma Devi, who was the muse of group-inquiry at its inception and continues to be to this day.

It wasn't until 1992 in Australia that I began to do Self-inquiry groups, naming the guided meditation and, later, the groups based on it, the Shiva Process. I saw these groups as the study and worship of Shiva or supreme Consciousness, but that did not prevent the early groups from being wild and woolly indeed.

There was an early debate about whether anger was good or detrimental for the group. I was alert to the arising of anger, and would immediately say, 'Anger has entered the room'. It was difficult to deal with. Once anger arose, a lot of work was required to overcome it. One person felt self-righteous, another felt hurt, another felt afraid.

Some of the early group members argued that this heightened the level of interest and excitement, and therefore was good. Certainly, anger brought more 'truth' to the process, but it was far more trouble than it was worth. As a result of this, I hit on the maxim, 'Tell the truth and don't get angry', based on a story from an Indian epic that expresses the need to find balance between the twin imperatives of truth and kindness. (I talk more about truth and kindness in Lecture 3.)

I love the practice of Self-inquiry. I am convinced that, along with deep meditation, it is the most valuable spiritual technique. A few years ago, during one of our retreats here in Mt Eliza, I gave a series of lectures on Self-inquiry. My plan was to do a comprehensive teaching on Self-inquiry, and later turn it into a book. During the editing process, I made the decision to keep the original integrity of the lecture format rather than create a textbook. My hope is that informality creates readability.

It soon became apparent to me that it is impossible to say everything there is about Self-inquiry. If inquiry is homologous with Consciousness, it is also infinite. A book cannot encompass the infinite, so I have tried to be content with communicating a *vision* of Self-inquiry. I hope the reader will open to it intuitively and even mystically.

Before we turn to the lectures, I should also say something more about Kashmir Shaivism. Many times I say, 'Shaivism says ...' or 'A Shaivite would say ...' or 'Kashmir Shaivism holds ...' Shaivism, like Vedanta, is what I call a philosophy of Consciousness. By that I mean that these two schools agree that there is essentially one substance in the universe, and that is Consciousness itself. While Vedanta and Kashmir Shaivism spend a lot of time and energy debating each other, in actual fact, their areas of agreement are much larger and more central than their areas of disagreement.

In contradistinction to these two, there is the dualistic philosophy of Samkhya, which has had many adherents in Indian spirituality, most notably the great yogi, Patanjali. Samkhya says that there are two, not one, independent substances in the universe: Consciousness and matter. Both are eternal and irreducible. The yogi of Samkhya feels that the conscious self has become contaminated by its engagement with matter and must be extricated. While I am philosophically in agreement with the point of view of the monistic philosophies of Consciousness, in practice, the Samkhyan approach is valuable.

Kashmir Shaivism says that Consciousness, the formless divine principle, contracts to become this universe, including human beings. Human beings suffer in separation from their source and then, through grace and yogic effort, return to it, discovering oneness with Consciousness. For a more detailed exploration of the philosophy and yoga of Kashmir Shaivism, see my book *Consciousness Is Everything*. From the perspective of Shaivism, Self-inquiry is nothing but the study of one's own consciousness. Understanding our own consciousness, we also understand universal Consciousness.

My own spiritual career has seen me spend years in India. I studied many an arcane text suffused with Sanskrit quotations and a highly specialised vocabulary. Hidden within that largely unavailable world, I found a timeless wisdom that would be exceedingly helpful in the contemporary West. I set myself the task of distilling and presenting it with a minimum of esoterica and foreign terminology.

The Shiva Process begins with simple questions and direct statements that anyone can understand. It uses these tools to reveal hidden feelings and motivations. If negative thoughts and feelings are repressed, they find a covert way to express themselves. There may be confusion, anger, panic or emotional discomfort without any obvious cause. Bringing them to light begins the process of resolution. The Shiva Process asks us to look at what we are feeling, to become conscious of the tensions that lie just outside of our normal awareness. As we turn inward, our internal conflicts and contradictions begin to dissolve and become balanced—even turning into creative and energising forces—as a natural consequence of deepening awareness.

ABOUT THIS BOOK

The book is in three sections. The first deals with personal inquiry, the inquiry practised within yourself during meditation. The second deals with group-inquiry, the form of inquiry practised in what I call Shiva Process groups. Self-inquiry is the generic term which includes all kinds of inquiry. Thus, both personal inquiry and group-inquiry are forms of Self-inquiry. The third section deals with both personal and group-inquiry, and views them through a new paradigm.

One cautionary note: *everyone* can profit from personal Self-inquiry, but one should learn the group process only from trained group leaders. There are many pitfalls and hazards in the group process that can be easily avoided with good training. Nonetheless, even if you don't practise group-inquiry, I think it will be profitable for you to read the section on it because that can only help your personal Self-inquiry and also your interactions. Along with personal inquiry and group-inquiry, there's a third type of Shiva Process Self-inquiry, and that is done in one-on-one private sessions with a Shiva Process facilitator (see Appendix I).

Accompanying the book is a CD in which a selection of inquiries are articulated. (See Appendix J for a summary of recorded inquiries.) To do personal inquiry, simply play Tracks 9 and 10 and inquiry will automatically happen. There are other inquiries designed to deal with areas of life (see Appendix D), and many more throughout to help access the Self.

To make the best use of this book, I suggest that you listen to Track 1, the Self-Inquiry Guided Chakra Meditation (Appendix E) and Track 2, the Healing Meditation (Appendix F) every day during the period when you read this book. Doing the practice in this way will illuminate aspects of the book which otherwise might seem abstract or unclear. Your inquiry will develop in a natural and organic manner.

A NOTE TO NON-SEEKERS

Dear Friends,

The Shiva Process does not require an esoteric philosophical or religious stance. You may not feel that you are a 'spiritual person' or have interest in spiritual matters, but you will have to admit that your mood and inner state are important to you. Doesn't it behove you to understand the laws of the mind and the emotions, which are the same for everyone, spiritual or not? It is likely that if you are reading this, you have already developed an interest in these matters.

You might not choose to avail yourself of G-*Statements* (that category of B-Statements associated with spiritual upliftment), but everyone needs to know about and use A- and B-Statements. It was a central intention of mine to find a spiritual method that used yogic insight without ethnic or cultic surroundings, even though I refer to Eastern sources in this book. You can use the method in this book to better understand the basic building blocks and inner laws of your inner world.

A NOTE TO SEEKERS

Dear Ones,

I respect that you probably have your own spiritual path. I'm not suggesting that the method described in this book should replace whatever practice you have found valuable and meaningful. Rather, I think Self-inquiry can help to complete the circle of your practice. As I've said, it arose spontaneously within me and had that effect on my own spiritual work.

Perhaps you meditate on pure Consciousness, on the witness, on thought-free awareness. In Shaivism, that is called the *shambhavopaya* method of pure Consciousness. In truth, it is part of Self-inquiry. You may already have found that life issues obtrude on your meditation and bring in unwanted thoughts and feelings. Self-inquiry gives you a method for resolving such issues, issues that even the greatest *jnani*, wise person, has to face.

Some of you may be reluctant to use inquiry in the way I describe here, fearing that it is too much about emotions and, therefore, merely psychological work. I don't think of inquiry that way. For me, it is about releasing tensions in the energy system. What is tension but a block in feeling? Tension is one way that negative emotion shows up. Where energy flows freely, there is no negative emotion and, in fact, there is liberation. Thus, Self-inquiry, at least in its Shiva Process form, includes all efforts to release tensions and blocks, leading to immersion in the conscious Self.

THE CONTAMINATED INNER SPACE: A NOTE ON SELF-INQUIRY

Finally, some general remarks on Self-inquiry. As I have said, the ancient Indian philosophy of Samkhya holds that a human individual is pure spirit, but because of ignorance has become contaminated by matter. Samkhya enjoins us to pull away from all material involvement and retreat into the purity of the Self. This is a useful, if incomplete, understanding. Our inner space in its purest form is free, clear and lucid. Later in the book, I will call this the 'clear space of good feeling'.

Self-inquiry is a method for dealing with the 'contaminated inner space', whether that contamination is caused by 'matter' or specifically by movements of fear and desire in regard to objects and other people. The inner space can be contaminated by confusion, by anger, by fear, by jealousy, by depression, by false subpersonalities, by painful memories; the list is long. Other people can metaphorically enter that inner space, where only the Self should exist, and cause confusion (see the section on *internal considering* in Lecture 5). True inquiry skilfully deals with contamination in any of its forms. It discovers blocks and restores flow.

PART I
PERSONAL INQUIRY

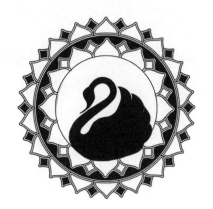

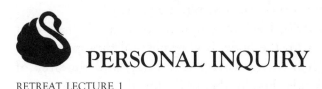 PERSONAL INQUIRY

All paths end in inquiry.
Why not pursue inquiry from the beginning?
Sri Ramana Maharshi

You are so blinded by what is personal, that you do not see the
universal. The blindness will not end by itself—it must be
undone skillfully and deliberately.
Sri Nisargadatta Maharaj

EVERY SPIRITUAL PATH, every yogic method, has a core practice. A mantra yogi always returns to his mantra. A *jnani* always returns to one noble thought. A devotee, a *bhakta*, always returns to the image of the beloved deity. In the same way, one who practises Self-inquiry always returns to the present moment and present experience.

In that spirit, let's become aware of our experience in this moment.

CONTEMPLATION: TASTING YOUR INNER WORLD

Close your eyes for a moment and look within. 'Taste' your inner world, becoming aware of areas of tension and also any areas in which the energy flows in a positive way. Your inquiry will always begin with this simple awareness. Your present awareness is the doorway to all deeper information and experience.

Self-inquiry is about unblocking the life force. If the life force is completely unblocked in all areas, a person becomes productive, well balanced and joyous. Blocks show up as tension, discomfort, pain or negative emotion in various places within the body.

Life can be described as having four major areas: the *body*—that is, everything to do with the body: health, physical fitness, diet and so on; *career*—which involves work and money; and the area of *relationships* of all kinds. Finally there is a fourth area, which can be called *spirituality*.

I had a board game called *Careers* when I was a teenager. You sought fame, fortune or happiness. Stars represented fame, $$$s represented fortune, and hearts represented happiness. You tried to attain your goal in each area, striving for 60 points, as I remember. You created your own formula with a lean towards fame, fortune or happiness as you valued them. When I create my version, I will make four categories: the body, career, relationship, and spirituality—I might call it *The God Game*.

Corresponding to the four areas of life are the four states of Consciousness. We know three of them well: waking, dream and deep sleep. Every day, we go through these three—we are awake for roughly two-thirds of the time, and then asleep for a third. Part of that sleep time is deep sleep, and part of that time is dreaming.

Beyond these three states, is *turiya*, a fourth state of Consciousness. It is a state of deep meditation or connectedness with the Self. Truly understood, this fourth state isn't a separate state, but involves contact with the Self. It actually underlies the other three. When we have done enough practice, when we have meditated well enough, that fourth state starts to penetrate or permeate the rest of our experience of life. Then, even while we are doing our normal daily business, we are in touch with that fourth state.

Great beings, yogis with high spiritual attainment, are always in an awakened state of Consciousness. Even while doing mundane things—talking about this, doing that, chatting about this, deciding that—they are centred in the Self. We first contact *turiya* in deep meditation, then, having discovered its qualities and its location, we bring it into, or discover it, in our waking life.

In the same way, like the state of *turiya*, spirituality is not a separate area. Of course, it is possible to think of your spirituality as a separate area. You could say, 'Now I am going to do my health; I'll do 20 push-ups. Now, I am going to do my career; I'll write some cheques. Now, I'll do my relationship; I'll send a bouquet of flowers or a text message'. And then you could say, 'Now I'll do my spirituality; I'll say my mantra for 20 minutes, or I'll meditate'. But compartmentalising it in that way shows a superficial understanding of spirituality. Spirituality underlies everything—it underlies all the other areas of life. If we bring spirituality into our career, we do better in our career, and if we bring it into our relationship, we do better in our relationship. Spirituality is the truth underlying all of life, in the same way that the *turiya* state underlies the waking, dream and deep-sleep states.

Self-inquiry can unblock these four areas of life. Essentially, it unblocks the spiritual area, which can then flow into the others. Our issues are always, finally, spiritual problems. Self-inquiry, as opposed to psychoanalysis or other methods, is remarkably direct. It always goes towards the target. You don't have to do years of analysis, dream analysis, free association and the like. In Self-inquiry, we look directly at what *is*—we see the block and undo it.

ONE SUBJECT AND MANY OBJECTS

When our attention is focused outside of ourselves, our unexamined belief is that the blocks and obstacles that arise in our life belong to the objects and events of the outer world. But along with living in a world filled with objects and other people, we live simultaneously in a second world: the inner world; the world of the Self.

Caught up in the charisma of outer objects and other people, it's easy to undervalue the importance of the inner world. Let's think about it for a moment:

- The capacity to question, to analyse and to understand is a property of the inner world and not the outer world.

- The capacity to suffer and to enjoy are powers of the inner world.

37

- The capacity to fear and to be heroic are powers of the inner world.

- The capacity to remember and also to forget are powers of the inner world.

- The capacity to love and to hate are powers of the inner world.

- The capacity to forgive, to bless and to feel blessed are powers of the inner world.

Blocks, too, actually belong to the inner world and not the outer world. Our emotional relationship to outer objects creates blocks. 'I want something that I can't have. I fear something that I can't avoid.' Desire and fear put us into a struggle with things as they are; a struggle that shows up as contraction in our inner world. Self-inquiry is meant to discover and release that contraction.

When I examine my experience here and now, I discover the odd fact that though there are many objects—infinite objects—in the universe, in my universe, there is only one subject. I believe that this remarkable fact of my reality is true of your reality as well: there is one subject in your universe and many objects. But since I cannot directly know *your* universe, let me stay with *my* universe. Since my earliest memory, there has been only one subject in my universe and many objects. As I sit here with you now, there is only one subject in my universe and many objects. That has been my total experience. And I expect, I am certain, that as long as I live, there will be one subject and many objects. When I die, there will be one subject and many objects.

This simple and directly perceived truth is rarely noticed, but well worth considering. No matter what happens in my world, in my universe, there is still only *me* and the rest of everything. I feel completely certain that this is true for you, too. This is a knowledge that should make us free. Nothing can affect that. Everything else is the details. It's just me and all the other objects.

Among the objects in my outer world, some are of a special kind because they seem likely to be subjects in their own universe. They appear to have interiority. I am speaking, of course, of other people and perhaps animals. The Shaivite masters held that the one subject of each of our personal universes is, in fact, the *same* subject. And that subject is Shiva or divine Consciousness. If we go inward far enough, we all get to the same place; we discover the same universal person, despite apparent differences.

The peculiarity of your inner world is that there is no one in it but you. Every other person, no matter how close to you, is still always and only an object in your universe. Your beloved can help you get dressed and drive you to work but they can never feel or think for you. No matter how ideal Ridge, Thorne and Brooke are, they can never merge with your subjectivity. Our thirst for relationship is really the desire to commune with the inner subject projected outside ourselves. The spiritual truth is that if we commune sufficiently with the one *in here*, then our connection with everyone else becomes perfect. Since there is no one else but me in my inner world and no one else but you in your inner world, no one but me or you will do Self-inquiry. And since the inner world holds the key to our right relationship to the outer world, Self-inquiry is in order.

UNBLOCKING SECOND FORCE

The Greek-Armenian mystic G. I. Gurdjieff taught that every event and experience in life is subject to three forces. His idea of the 'Law of Three' illumines the practice of Self-inquiry. *First force* is the initiating force or creative force; *second force* is the block or resistance that all creativity encounters; *third force* is the solution that enables you to overcome second force. It is grace.

The German philosopher Hegel said essentially the same thing: first there is the *thesis*, which creates its own *antithesis*, and together they produce a new *synthesis*. This Hegelian Dialectic is a powerful construction. Hegel and later Marx used it to explain major developments in human social evolution. Gurdjieff demonstrates that it is useful in individual evolution as well.

In Gurdjieff's system, first force has to do with the inner world because it is in the inner world that desire and creativity exist. Look around you at every manufactured object in the room. Each one of them took birth, first of all, in someone's inner world. Someone said,

'I'd like to make this. I want to invent that'. Perhaps this is why the most intimate inner space is called the *causal* world. In the inner world of awareness, there is a great deal of freedom. A person can think any kind of thought at any time.

Next we come to second force, which is related to the outer world, although it also shows up within us as some form of disharmony. It's easy to have an idea in the inner world; it's quite another thing to bring that idea to fruition. The outer world is material and resistant. It takes effort and varying degrees of struggle to realise an idea in physical reality. When an idea encounters matter, a tension arises. A third force is required in the form of know-how or inspiration, an insight or technique, or even money. It enables the original vision to be manifested.

Think of Michelangelo's desire to create a statue of David as first force. The intransigence of the block of marble is second force, and his sculptural skill is third force. Second force shows up within us as the feeling of tension and frustration we experience when it is difficult or impossible to get what we want. If we pay close attention, we can locate the feeling as a tension in the navel or elsewhere within the body. It is precisely this experience of second force as inner feeling that is the main focus of our inquiry. Second force arises where spirit or Consciousness meets matter. It reflects the emotional strain that spirit experiences operating in material reality. Spiritually considered, second force is not outside of us, but within us. Through inquiry and understanding, we search for ways to diminish it or remove it. The material realm remains just as stubborn as ever, but we learn to negotiate it or to accept it peacefully.

Everyone in the world, not just yogis, deals with the problem of second force. It is common to experience a feeling of limitation that cuts across a number of areas of life. We can't stamp our will on reality sufficiently to achieve satisfaction and peace. All the normal strategies of life—seeking a good relationship, getting more money, improving health, seeking fame and honour—are all strategies to overcome second force and bring in third force.

A yogi doesn't despise these strategies, but knows they are limited. There exists a much wider range of strategies for attaining third force:

spiritual strategies and methods. Yogis do not say, 'Give up your relationships and hate money'; they say, 'Pursue your goals', but add the wisdom and broader context that meditation and spiritual inquiry provide.

It is crucial to see that we ourselves create the experience of tension, or second force, within ourselves by our emotional relationship to the outer world. Specifically, we desire and we fear. Maurice Nicoll, one of Gurdjieff's best interpreters, emphasised becoming aware in first force. Simply put, he meant that we should know what we want in every situation. If we have hidden our true motives from ourselves, we don't understand why second force arises. Let's explore this through inquiry.

INQUIRY: BECOMING AWAKE IN FIRST FORCE

Close your eyes. Think of a situation in your life in which you feel blocked. Locate the block in your body and be aware of it as second force. Second force cannot exist unless you are producing first force, some desire that is frustrated. Inquire into the feeling and ask, 'What do I really want here?' Articulate it to yourself clearly. Notice the effect on your inner world.

Recently, while preparing a series of lectures on the teachings of the Buddha, I came to the remarkable conclusion that the Buddha's four noble truths are simply a different way of talking about the three forces. It's not surprising that the Buddha's path can be expressed in terms of the three forces because ultimately spirituality is about undoing second force and arriving at Consciousness. The Buddha's four noble truths could be summarised as follows:

1.   There is suffering.

2.   Suffering has a cause (desire).

3.   Suffering can be overcome.

4.   There is an eightfold path to end suffering.

Using the three forces, the Buddha's truths would go something like this:

1.   There is second force (tension, block).

2.   Second force is caused by first force (desire).

3.   Second force can be overcome by third force.

4.   Third force can be brought into all areas of your life through an eightfold methodology.

The Buddha's eightfold path is designed to decrease tension and bring flow into career, relationships, conversation and the inner life. These different aspects of living each have their own methodology, hence, right view, right speech, right livelihood, right meditation and so on. The 'right' method decreases second force and increases grace.

HARMONISING THINKING, FEELING AND DOING

We are thinking-feeling-doing creatures. We think, we feel and we do. These three characteristic and essential activities can be brought into balance by means of effective Self-inquiry. According to whether we favour thinking, feeling or doing, we fit into one of three main types.

Some of us are thinkers who don't feel much. We think and think. Maybe we don't do much either. Others are 'feelers'. Everything is a feeling or an emotional experience. In such a person, the thinking process might not be very developed. This type has a problem with doing because they tend to be overwhelmed by feeling. A third type is the doer. Such a person doesn't think or feel very much. At the slightest impulse, they are off and running—maybe in the wrong direction. They only learn they are going in the wrong direction when they run into a wall. Then they start over. You may not be able to work out your own type right away, but you might recognise a friend's type.

Self-inquiry harmonises and brings together the three modalities. We run into trouble if thought and feeling become too far apart. Some of the greatest atrocities in the world came about because thought and feeling split apart. Someone may love their own ideas but not notice that the feeling accompanying them is horrific and even murderous. If you go too far out just on thinking, you can get out of touch with your humanity. I'm thinking, of course, of monsters like Hitler.

On the other hand, if feeling is emphasised to the detriment of intellect and action, there is no stability. Such a person goes up and down all the time. We need to integrate thought and feeling. Real inquiry does that, bringing thought and feeling together. It is important to become aware of our underlying feeling. When we act, whatever feeling we act from affects the outcome. If there is anger inside of us and we think and act out of that anger, we do things that later, when we are not so angry, we regret. It is important to understand the motive behind each of our actions. Inquiry gets us in touch with that. Inquiry joins thought to feeling and then it helps put things into action.

When thought and feeling merge, the resultant is what I call 'wisdom power'. To understand wisdom power, think about what is involved in giving up smoking. A person has the idea 'I should stop smoking'. That's a good idea and we could say it has wisdom in it. But do they have the power to actually do it? If 100 people want to stop smoking, only a few of them actually succeed. The ones who succeed have wisdom power; that is, they have the will or emotion that brings their idea to fruition. In Shaivite terms, they have not only *jnana*, knowledge, but also *iccha*, will.

It is obvious that the dissociation of thought and feeling is an epidemic in our culture. There are two kinds of problems that arise. When thought is strong but emotion is weak, the person is ineffectual. When emotion is strong but thought is weak, the person is effective at doing many foolish things. Wisdom power comes when thought and feeling merge.

The inner world consists precisely of thought and feeling. Thought and feeling are two sides of the same coin: when thought is positive, feeling is positive; when thought is negative, feeling is negative. When thought and feeling are brought together, then a sort of alchemy happens, and understanding and energy expand. A corollary to Gurdjieff's three forces is that when two principles are brought together, a third thing flowers. When awareness is joined to the breath, for example, a meditator notices an unmistakeable inner quickening.

A sage or a realised being is perfectly integrated in these three areas—thinking, feeling and doing are all harmonious. Nonetheless, every great sage has their unique personality. Some are more devotional, like the 19th-century sage Sri Ramakrishna; some more intellectual, like the 10th-century Shaivite sage Abhinavagupta, and some more vital, like Baba Muktananda. What happens is, their most deficient area has been strengthened during the course of their *sadhana*. Baba is a good example. He was exceptionally strong and operational in each of the three areas. He was a great *bhakta* of his Guru, and also a wonderful writer and profound student of the scriptures. Still, his amazing vitality was always the most immediately apparent thing about him. My hunch, based on intuition and his own testimony, is that the key to Baba's later attainment was the explosion of his devotional nature, which happened when he opened to his Guru. Formerly, that was his weakest link, and its opening balanced Baba and made him great.

PERSONAL AND IMPERSONAL

Real inquiry marries the head and heart. Thought, which has been wandering in its own bloodless world, feeding on itself, is connected to feeling. And like two wires touched together, a spark of energy occurs. Inquiry is also the conjunction of the personal and impersonal. The ancient yogic paths emphasised the impersonal. They insisted that this world does not exist and you are not a separate person. In Indian culture, you are expected to fit into your particular role in life, your caste, your stage of life. You are to do your duty and any deviation is tantamount to insanity. The single social option to the non-conformist is the possibility of renouncing the world and heading off to the Himalayas to be a wandering monk.

In the West, on the contrary, we hear everywhere the cry, 'What about me?' We are obsessed with our individuality and our individual expression. The West is totally focused on the person. In India, the yoga is impersonal, connected to the highest truth, caring little for the person. One must maintain an appropriate silence about personal problems and simply do *sadhana* and one's duty.

Yoga says that within each person, in the subtle body, are seven yogic centres, seven chakras, which have to do with different aspects of life. The three lower chakras govern the physical life; the heart chakra is the locus of emotional life; the fifth chakra, in the throat, has to do with communication; the third eye, the sixth chakra, is the place of intellect and higher wisdom. Here we have insights and visions but we are still within the personal realm. When you go beyond the sixth chakra to the seventh, at the crown of the head, you contact a different aspect of yourself. It is transpersonal; the dimension of the impersonal Self.

Western psychology was traditionally unaware of this dimension. In the past 30 years, however, a 'transpersonal psychology' has developed, acknowledging that divine, impersonal aspect. Jung knew of it but Freud did not. It exists within all of us, represented by the seventh chakra. What should we make of this knowledge of a higher reality? The first impulse is to try to override the person with the impersonal. A noble goal, but significantly difficult to attain. I tried to achieve it: I threw myself on the altar of impersonality again and again. Each time, the person returned. That the higher power does exist is beyond doubt, but the mystical play between the personal and impersonal has to be discovered.

My Guru seemed to me to be a man who was in cosmic awareness. He was always connected to the Self, and never unconnected. Yet, he was also very much a person. He wasn't like some of the mind-borne 'holy men': 'Hello my son, at last you have come . . .' He wasn't like that at all. He was completely vibrant and immediate and totally himself—to an alarming degree, in fact. He was a unique combination of the personal and the impersonal. He was a force of nature, all right. Like a stone rolling down a hill, and loving it.

Self-inquiry connects the personal with the impersonal. It respects the person. It doesn't try to kill the person, but it also acknowledges the transpersonal. It seeks connectedness so that the person flowers within the impersonal and discovers the impersonal within. A life without the impersonal is dry and empty. You want the universe to flow towards your personal advantage, but, alas, the universe is indifferent. What chance does the poor little person have? The whole universe is arranged to frustrate or be indifferent to your desires. There is no joy in being merely a person.

Sometimes we feel a part of something bigger than ourselves. It might be a political movement, or even a crowd cheering for a team at a football game. It is a rewarding and liberating feeling. Our individuality dissolves in the group, and, at the same time, participates actively. But when the event is over or we leave the group for some reason, we feel a kind of loss—we've returned to the merely personal.

Such an experience is only temporary, but it is a taste of something real and intrinsic to our true Self. We are actually part of something greater, and when we live in harmony with it, our stress and fear fade away.

Through the process of inquiry, we recognise the dynamism running through us. We become liberated from doubt and concern when we no longer try to hold the universe at bay, but surrender to it, and welcome it. Our actions become effective and powerful, because they are aligned with this great impersonal process. And we have the delightful experience of playing our part in a larger drama.

PRATYABHIJNAHRIDAYAM SUTRA 11:
THE ESOTERIC FIVE PROCESSES

Self-inquiry arose within me as a spontaneous effect of being in my Guru's presence. Later, after developing the Shiva Process method, I became aware that it reflected many of the principles of Kashmir Shaivism. A scholarly study entitled *The Shaivite Underpinnings of the Shiva Process* could be written and it would be interesting, but that is not my purpose here. I will, however, look at one of the sutras of Shaivism, *Pratyabhijnahridayam* Sutra 11, which is the Shaivite teaching perhaps most integral to our method of inquiry.

Pratyabhijnahridayam was written by the Shaivite sage Kshemaraja in the 10th century, and is one of the Kashmir Shaivite texts we have in English. It has only 20 sutras (aphorisms) and is particularly user-friendly. *Pratyabhijnahridayam* means *The Heart of the Doctrine of Self-*

Recognition. As the title suggests, the text centres on recognition of the true Self.

Before speaking of Kshemaraja's 11th sutra, about the 'esoteric five processes', I have to first describe two other sets of five processes, 'the universal five processes' and 'the personal five processes'. Shaivism says that God or supreme Consciousness performs five actions, and so do we. The first three are *creation*, *sustainment* and *destruction*. These three are embodied in the Hindu trinity of Brahma, Vishnu and Shiva. God creates the universe, He sustains it for a while, and then He destroys it. We also create things, we sustain them for a while, and then we (or time) destroy them.

Everything undergoes this cycle in the world: a being is born, lives for a while and then dissolves. God, or, if you prefer, Mother Nature or universal Consciousness, creates, sustains and destroys. In our inner world—inside our minds—we do the same: we create a thought, we hold it for a while, and then it disappears. An emotion comes up, it stays for a while, it disappears—we create, we sustain, we dissolve.

The final two processes or actions are *concealment* and *grace*. Concealment is a universal principle, which is the same as maya or the great illusion. It creates separation, estrangement and ignorance. In Gurdjieff's terms, it is second force. Grace is the other universal process and it creates oneness, harmony, illumination and peace. In Gurdjieff's terms, it is third force. We know concealment and grace inside ourselves particularly well. Whenever you feel alienated, miserable and unhappy, you are experiencing concealment. And when you feel harmonious and happy, you are experiencing grace.

Our lives move between these two. When we experience concealment, we always want to move towards grace, though we might not know how. Grace is not only a thunderbolt the Guru throws at you so that your *kundalini* awakens and you jump and leap. Grace is there in everything—in a feeling of harmony, in a feeling of love, in a feeling of peace—under all circumstances.

Notice that the language Shaivism uses shows a definite leaning towards grace. When we say a thing is 'concealed', we hint that it is present, though hidden. In the same way, grace is always there, though sometimes hidden.

WHERE THE RUBBER MEETS THE ROAD

Thus, five processes unfold on the cosmic level (the outer world), and a parallel five processes take place on the personal level (the inner world); the macrocosm and microcosm. In the 11th sutra, the text cites a third group—the esoteric five processes. This is where the rubber meets the road. It is the point of impact. Spiritually, where the rubber meets the road is *now*. The rubber meets the road in the present moment. Right now and right now and right now again. This is where spirituality really takes place. The past is gone; right now is the spiritual moment. The esoteric five processes are about how we live in every second, how we interface with our world in every moment. And this is also what Self-inquiry is fundamentally about.

Kshemaraja says in *Pratyabhijnahridayam* Sutra 11:

> [The esoteric five processes consist of] manifesting, relishing, experiencing as Self, settling of the seed, and dissolution.

Here is the substance of what he means in practical terms. Let's begin with the moment you see something, you perceive something. This is the creation of that object for you *(manifesting)*. Then, as you keep it in your field of attention, you are sustaining it *(relishing)*. When you don't see it any more, you've destroyed it—you've dissolved it *(dissolution)*. You hear something, you sustain it for a while and then it disappears. For our purposes, what is really interesting is the discussion of grace and concealment, the last two processes.

Kshemaraja writes (loosely translated) in the commentary of *Pratyabhijnahridayam*:

> When we withdraw ourselves from a sensory experience, and that experience leaves various negative *samskaras* or impressions (of doubt, etc.), then that negative feeling is bound to rise up again at some future time, and in this way, the real nature of the Self is concealed.

When we experience something in the course of living, the experience lasts for a while and then it ends. We withdraw from our engagement with it. If the experience was accompanied by a negative emotion (like doubt, but we can include other emotions, such as fear or anger), then that very emotion will energise the memory of the experience and cause it to reappear later.

If, for example, you enter a bank, see the bank teller and cash a cheque, such an encounter is not fraught with emotion. Well, for some of us, maybe everything is fraught, but this is essentially a neutral encounter. We 'create' the teller, we are with the teller, and then we move off and we have a clean feeling. We don't usually say, 'Goodness, that was clean'. We simply go about our business and there is no *samskara* or tendency; nothing has been created that is going to rise up again.

However, suppose the teller does something that makes us angry. When we leave, that anger is still with us. It is held inside us. It might come out later in the day directed at other people. Or it might create a *samskara*, so that every time we go into a bank, we feel it by association. Or the poor teller might innocently awaken a *samskara* that lies hidden within us. The teller reminds us of someone in our past, and positive— or negative—associations well up. Perhaps the ATM is the safe alternative.

The crucial moment arrives after an action is completed. Did we live it cleanly or was it accompanied by negative or positive feeling? The key in this whole process, where the rubber meets the road, is emotion. Let's say you get angry, and you walk away from that encounter knowing 'I am angry'. If you are not a yogi, what you do then is offload that anger on someone as soon as you can, probably a suitably weak person. You can abuse that person, or be mean to your intimates or attack Swamiji. That is unconsciously acting out of anger.

But if you are interested in your inner process, if you are trying to attain freedom and truth, then you want to act responsibly. You know that you got angry and you feel it as a contamination. It feels bad and you want to get rid of it and you also want to make sure that it doesn't return later.

Moment to moment, we encounter the world. Things happen. We react to what is said and done. Perhaps we react in a tense way, in an angry way, in a separative way, in a confused way. As we interact with the world, we withdraw out of fear or we engage out of desire. Everything that happens is recorded within us as conscious or unconscious memory. Our state is affected, our experience is affected, and our point of view is affected.

Properly done, inquiry tunes our awareness to these interactions. We observe how we interface with our world. And we have to try, if we are yogis, to keep it clean. It is not good enough to be filled with rage and then get drunk. In a sense, the way of alcohol is a yoga, and the yogis of that way are also trying to get rid of second force and negative emotion. I don't have to tell you why that method has glaring shortcomings. We have to develop more appropriate means. Through wisdom, through inquiry, through meditative practice, we reduce or eliminate second force.

Where the rubber meets the road, it is best to surrender, to say 'yes', to not resist. Then we experience harmony and oneness. When we can't surrender and can't give assent, then we need to practise and be careful and aware. Sutra 11 focuses on how experience impacts us and the practice we need when we can't give our perfect 'yes'. The most challenging experiences always come about through other people. Other people are heaven and they are also hell. It is hard to get angry at a stone, but it is easy to get angry at another person. Another person is an object who is a subject in their own universe, as we are. And that uniquely raises the intensity of our interactions.

HATHAPAKA AND ALAMGRASA

So, what means do we have at our disposal to keep our interactions clean?

Kshemaraja writes (again, freely translated):

> If a yogi experiences the after-effect of an encounter and then holds it inwardly and burns it to sameness with the fire of Consciousness by the process of *hathapaka* and by the device of *alamgrasa*, then by bringing about perfection, he enters the state of grace.

The idea of 'burning to sameness with the fire of Consciousness' is one of the most important teachings in *Pratyabhijnahridayam*. *Hathapaka* and *alamgrasa* are not specific techniques—they are generic. They are powerful yogic methods of releasing negative emotion. Indeed, if you have the ability to get rid of anger by some technique, then you go into a state of grace or harmony or peace.

Hathapaka is a fiery and forceful method, and *alamgrasa* is a gradual method of assimilation. In yoga and in inquiry, the most important thing is your intuition. If you do regular inquiry, your intuition develops. Good tennis players have worked on technique. They know how to get their weight across and hit the backhand. But in play, every ball has a different flight. Every shot is different. They have to respond to each ball creatively and intuitively in the moment.

Similarly, we do have to develop our yogic technique, but in each moment we respond situationally. We have to bring our whole awareness into play. If we are gathering wool, if we are elsewhere engaged or lost in negative emotion, we won't be able to bring our full humanity and our wisdom power to bear. We have to be very present, like a flame, like a fire, and deal with everything as it arises.

The Shaivite scholar Jaideva Singh says that there are two ways in which experience can be 'burned to sameness' with the Self. They are *shanti-prasama* and *hathapaka-prasama*. *Prasama* means bringing to oneness. *Shanti-prasama* is a gradual and peaceful bringing to oneness or merging in the Self, while *hathapaka-prasama* is swift and energetic.

Hatha here implies strong effort. Some yogic methods work slowly and peacefully, while others, characterised by strong emotions like will, disgust or anger, work immediately. Baba used to say, 'If you have to be angry, then be angry at your anger'. Non-dual philosophy, the point of view that all is one, says that although objects appear to be outside of the subject, they are actually *within* the subject; that is, within Consciousness. The yogis on the path of wisdom gradually, or all at once, see everything, both outside and inside, as the reflection of their own Self.

When an experience is completely assimilated to Consciousness (burned to sameness), the Shaivites call it *alamgrasa*. *Alam* means fully, when no impression or seed remains, and *grasa* means swallowing. Thus, *alamgrasa* is a full swallowing of impressions. We swallow the whole experience. Normally, if we have an experience that gets us angry, we dramatise it and drag it out. We tell this one and we tell that one. Then we write a letter. Then we proclaim it to everyone and in doing so we give it more life; we increase its hold on us. This is the opposite of fully swallowing the experience.

We often refer to 'swallowing our anger', meaning to repress it. This is not the sense in *alamgrasa*. We also talk about being swallowed by anger or some other emotion, in the sense of being consumed by it, overwhelmed by it, or transformed by it. This is more the sense of 'swallowing' in *alamgrasa*, except it is the other way around: we accept, absorb and assimilate the experience. A character in one of John Updike's stories says, 'The world is the host, it must be chewed'.

In an Indian myth, the ocean was poisoned, threatening everything. Only Shiva could save the world. He drank the whole ocean. Because He was a great yogi, He could take the poison, drink it, and hold it within Himself. His throat turned blue and as a consequence He is called the Blue-Throated One, *Neelakantha*. Shiva was able to hold all the poison in the universe within Himself. Then, through *alamgrasa*, He digested it within, returned to peace, and the world was saved. By contrast, if we take a little poison, absorb a bad feeling or a bad vibration, we cry out in agony.

It is a great yogic and moral quality to be able to hold the negative, to contain it. When you are really angry, you know you are likely to do or say something you will regret. Instead, you sit down and you contain it. You work with it, and through inner methods, you get to a place of peace with it. When you sat down to meditate you were furious and when you stood up after 20 minutes or an hour, you were peaceful. It is a real spiritual triumph. This is *alamgrasa*.

It is not repression. A repressed emotion still exists as a seed ready to sprout at some unexpected time in some unexpected manner. *Alamgrasa* dissolves the transitory experience or emotion in persistent awareness. Awareness is always immediate. It is right now. Lingering resentment and the like are historical. They are about something that happened in the past.

To become a master of the five processes is to be in control of our manifestation, to be able to sort out our emotions within ourselves. If we spread our negative emotions everywhere, we create endless chains of complexity and misery. This is precisely what the esoteric five processes tell us: we create karma when we offload our negative emotions onto others. We go through the same things again and again. It is much better to learn to practise forbearance and strive to find our way back to peace.

The inner or yogic criterion of truth is the feeling of harmony. Truth always has a feeling of harmony and peace. When you are in a state of agitation and suffering, it means you have not arrived at truth. The Self, which is truth, is also a state of love, peace and perfection. That is your inner standard. It is not an objective standard. Even if the whole world says something, you know inside whether it is true or not by your inner feeling. It is an inner knowing. Too often, we don't listen to that inner feeling; instead, we listen to what everybody else says. One of the things that happens when we go deeper in inquiry and meditation is that we listen to our own feeling.

In the next lecture, I will talk about a technology by which we can control our manifestation. Later on, I will speak about the specific forms of *hathapaka* and *alamgrasa* we use in the Shiva Process method of Self-inquiry.

QUESTIONS AND ANSWERS

MERGING LOVE AND WISDOM

Question: I'm wondering if I'm more suited to the path of devotion than the path of Self-inquiry. Could you comment on these two approaches?

Swamiji: Indian philosophy has always recognised these two paths. In the path of devotion, a particular form of God is supremely attractive and the yogi is drawn towards the goal by means of love. The traditional path of wisdom is characterised, not by attraction, but by negation. Yogis divest themselves of what is inessential or wrong.

Nisargadatta Maharaj used to point out that both of these are moods which alternate. He thought that sometimes a person is attracted to the truth and sometimes repelled by the false. Both movements should be honoured and when the mood arises, you should go with it.

Self-inquiry, in its most common form, is an example of the path of negation. The Self is eternally present but obscured by ignorance, blocks and the negative movements of the mind. Nothing has to be done to draw closer to the Self, we simply have to get rid of the obscuring elements, which are like clouds in front of the sun. When that process is complete, the Self stands revealed. In the path of wisdom, Self-inquiry is the main instrument.

So, even if you have a leaning towards devotion, both approaches are valid and a well-rounded practice will include both of them. You will discover that Shiva Process Self-inquiry is designed to include both.

WHAT IS CONSCIOUSNESS?

Question: You keep referring to Consciousness. What is Consciousness?

Swamiji: Consciousness is not different from awareness. And individual consciousness is the same as universal Consciousness, the way that a puddle of water is not different from the ocean. Notice the faculty through which you experience yourself as alive and aware, here and now. That is Consciousness. By means of Consciousness, you see and hear, think and feel, love and hate. In short, you experience everything in life.

Consciousness is fluid. Within Consciousness, however, there is a capacity to create structure by means of language. Eventually, this structuring element becomes the material universe. Matter is relatively rigid and stable. The yogi of inquiry tries to break down structures and create flow. The more we flow in Consciousness, the more joyous and easy is our experience of life. Right now, Consciousness is speaking to you through me, and Consciousness is listening to me in you.

RELEASING BLOCKS

Question: Why do we have blocks?

Swamiji: That's too big a question. It's like asking, 'Why is there suffering?' But on a practical level, a block is a cathexis of energy. Energy which is free-flowing becomes bound in an idea or feeling. So, a block is a thought-feeling complex that contains a lot of energy. If you learn how to unblock a block, you learn how to release energy in almost the same way nuclear fission does.

We create blocks by wrong or limited thinking, by being caught in the ego or in desire, and we release blocks by right thought and right action. When we come to the right perspective on a thing, person or event, our tension releases and we are flooded with good energy. This is why an intelligent person does inquiry to release blocks.

A block shows the presence of second force. Normally, we feel that outer circumstances (karma, fate, other people) work against our getting what we want. A person who does inquiry discovers that second force is generated inwardly. This is quite shocking. But think of it this way—the external universe is simply what it is. It doesn't do anything to you. On the other hand, you (we) have all kinds of demands. When the indifferent universe doesn't meet them, we feel blocked.

So, who is doing what to whom? There was once a student of my Guru who was creating a lot of second force in a particular context. He was battered and confused, so Baba took him out of that situation. After a while, Baba decided to send him back into the fray. The fellow was terrified. Baba pointed to a shoe rack filled with shoes. He said, 'Be like those shoes, just lie there and do nothing'. Following that advice, the student did much better on his return. And he discovered that it was his own internal doings that created all his problems.

SUFFERING AND TRANSFORMATION

Question: Hearing about Shiva swallowing the poison reminds me of Christ's sacrifice on the cross. Could you speak about that?

Swamiji: Christian theology says Jesus died for our sins. He certainly underwent frightful suffering in many different ways. One possible understanding is that by being able to hold the full reality of the world in the form of extreme and ultimate suffering, he performed a transforming act. It is said, 'Everyone has a cross to bear'. The cross is second force. It is the cross of matter. The cross has been explained as symbolic of the intersection of matter and spirit.

We are spiritual creatures, full of Consciousness and love, and yet we are stuck in matter and we are confused by it. So much second force arises; so many blocks and difficulties. This material world is the arena of transformation. This is where you have to get it right, or not. It is a great test, a great struggle. Christ, like all the sages, stands for the triumph of the spirit in the midst of the limitations of the physical world; the triumph of Self over ego.

THE TRANSCENDENTAL AND THE PERSONAL

Question: I'm used to meditating to experience the transcendental Self. I'm afraid that Self-inquiry will emphasise the person and make me more neurotic.

Swamiji: The Shiva Process assumes 'You are Shiva'. Its basic stance is that you are not the neurotic, hung-up person you fear or believe you are. You need a new understanding to unblock the blocked areas of your life and your Shiva nature will manifest.

Moreover, the Shiva Process has faith that this new understanding is always available to you. The Shiva Process is a technique to find that understanding. Its real focus is not on your personhood but on your higher Self, and every participant can learn to access it.

Question: Aren't negative emotions good for anything?

Swamiji: As a card-carrying Shaivite, I have to be committed to the view that everything is Shiva, don't I? So, negative emotions have to be Shiva, too. And if you read the Puranas, Shiva Himself got angry, *really* angry.

My observation about negative emotions is that they are a form of energy that is good for something. Sadness, irritation, loneliness, anger—they are all tools for something.

If God puts a hammer in my hand, there must be a nail around here somewhere. Maybe it is not always clear what they are good for. But they are at least always good as a starting point for inquiry, as a spur to investigation.

How much great art is based on a masterly use of negative emotions? 'My baby done left me ... Seems my blues is all I own.' Why is that uplifting? The universe of Consciousness is very mysterious. It takes a yogic squint to change from indulging the emotion to recognising that it is something for you to observe, to discard or to relish. But you can only do this from the perspective of the Self.

USING INQUIRY FOR YOUR CAREER

Question: You mentioned that inquiry can be useful in all areas of life. I'm particularly interested in its application to the corporate sphere. Could you comment on that?

Swamiji: Yes, it's very effective in that arena and I know a few people who are doing that kind of coaching work. Again, Gurdjieff's paradigm gives us a valuable clue. Remember he talked about the three forces: initiating (first force), resisting (second force) and resolving (third force). Let's call first force 'purpose'. All business ventures begin with a purpose, an aim, a vision. As soon as the purpose is expressed, second force arises: 'obstacle.' Obstacle is also reality because only God can manifest His desire instantly; the rest of us have to actually work for it.

Every business aim has numerous technical difficulties to overcome. These will show up as tension within the body of the executive or executive group. By processing and releasing that tension, we bring in third force, which is the force of 'resolution'. Maybe we have to think outside the box or modify the aim to bring it more in harmony with what is actually possible, or maybe we find a new source of capital.

The interesting thing is that once again, the second force has shown up as tension in the inner world and releases when the appropriate outer world solution is found. Block becomes flow, and vision becomes manifestation.

Inquiry in the corporate sphere is somewhat different from inquiry in the personal sphere. While the goal of every kind of Shiva Process Self-inquiry is to translate knowing into action, the emphasis on action is even more critical in the corporate sphere. In that world, how a person feels is (lamentably or not) far less important than a question like 'What should I do and how should I do it?' Shiva Process is easily adapted to this emphasis.

MASTERING THE FIVE PROCESSES

Question: Do you have any practical hints about becoming a master of the five processes?

Swamiji: If you become adept at inquiry, you become a master of the five processes. Then you become aware of how every event and encounter impacts you. Since you are the only subject of your universe, you create, sustain and destroy your own experience. Moment to moment, you experience either grace or concealment. Grace is marked by expansion and upliftment, while concealment is marked by contraction and pain.

Advanced meditators can tune in immediately to their present experience. But a good thing that anyone can do is to review their day each evening. With eyes closed, ask yourself if there were any experiences today where doubt arose or where you experienced a jarring moment. You will more than likely find a few. Examine them contemplatively. Did you handle the feeling in the moment, or not? If the feeling is still with you, try to find a way to 'burn it to sameness'.

In the beginning stages of inquiry, it is enough to simply be aware of those jarring moments without trying to do anything about them.

TRACK 3. INQUIRY: REVIEWING YOUR DAY

Close your eyes. Review the day in sections. Think about the morning, the afternoon, the evening.

- Did your emotions shift and change during the day?

- Did you have an emotional reaction to any event or encounter?

- Particularly regarding negative experiences, did you handle the emotion immediately or not?

- Did the emotion affect later events during the day?

- Is the feeling still with you?

- What did you need to do at the time to shift your experience?

- What do you need to do now to shift your experience?

SUMMARY

- Self-inquiry seeks to unblock all areas of life: health, career, relationship and spirituality.

- Blocks are tensions in our inner world.

- Desire and fear create blocks.

- There is one subject and many objects.

- First force initiates, second force resists, third force enables.

- Second force as blocked inner feeling is the main focus of inquiry.

- Right method increases third force.

- Self-inquiry harmonises our thinking, feeling and doing.

- Wisdom power is where thought and feeling merge.

- Everything undergoes five processes: creation, sustainment, dissolution, concealment and grace.

- Concealment is the universal principle of separation.

- Grace is the universal principle of oneness.

- Our encounters in life are marked by emotion.

- Our negative reactions are stored inside and may reappear later.

- A yogi burns negative reactions to sameness with Consciousness.

- Truth has a feeling of harmony and peace.

- Self-inquiry is the main instrument in the wisdom path, yet it includes devotion.

- Shiva Process Self-inquiry focuses on the higher Self.

- Emotions are starting points for inquiry.

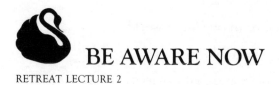 **BE AWARE NOW**

RETREAT LECTURE 2

*Inquiry (vichara) is the first and foremost step to be taken.
When vichara continues ... the 'I' thought becomes clearer for
inspection. The source of 'I' is the Heart–the final goal.*
Sri Ramana Maharshi

*Inquiry (the second gate-keeper to liberation) should be
undertaken by an intelligence that has been purified by a
close study of the scripture, and this inquiry should be
unbroken ... By such inquiry the intelligence becomes keen
and is able to realise the Supreme.*
Yoga Vashishta

THE ESOTERIC FIVE processes tell us to pay close attention to our
reactions as we engage with the world. 'Engagement with the world'
refers particularly to our encounters with other people. 'Did I get angry?
Did I feel jealous? Was I greedy? Was I fearful? What emotion arose in
that encounter?' If we don't deal with that, if we don't digest it properly,
it is stored inside as a *samskara*. Then it becomes a tendency, it builds
up and manifests later.

Real Self-inquiry requires minute awareness of everything that
happens. If it seems like a big job to be present to everything moment
to moment for the rest of your life, then I have a simpler alternative.
Be present now. Be aware now. Forget about all the times you weren't
aware, and certainly don't worry about all the times in the future

where you might perhaps not be aware. It's a terrible burden for your mind to think about all your future spiritual struggles, how you'll have to conquer ignorance every moment ad infinitum. Reduce the task to simply waking up in this moment. Just be present now. Whenever you remember to be present, become present, be aware. And if you can do that now, you'll be ready to handle the next moment when it arises. You'll feel a lot less neurotic.

THE QUESTION

In Sanskrit, Self-inquiry is *atma vichara*. *Atma* is Self, *vichara* is inquiry or investigation. When we talk about any kind of inquiry, we are talking about using questions to obtain knowledge. By the study and practice of Self-inquiry, I developed a real respect for the simple question. What is a question? A question is a technique by which Consciousness is focused. It is, therefore, a meditative device. If I ask you a question like 'What colour is that object?' then out of all the multiplicity of the universe, the many things and possibilities, by means of one swift remark, you bring all your attention to bear on that object and its colour. And what colour is it? The boys all think it's red, but the girls think it's mauve or puce or something. What is it? It's fuchsia or tangerine.

A question implies an answer. A question and an answer are two things that once were joined, but now are split apart. In higher Consciousness, knowledge is whole, but as Consciousness steps down, doubt or ignorance separates the question from its answer. The question is the pathway to an answer. When a question is asked, it rejoins itself to the answer. If you find the question, the answer is also there, or at least not far away. When you ask a spiritual question you may feel you are far from the spiritual goal, but, in truth, you are quite near it. If spiritual questions arise in your mind with any degree of frequency, they define you as a 'spiritual person'. Most people don't ask spiritual questions at all. The questions you ask yourself tell you everything about the life you lead.

There is a Cameroon proverb that says, if you ask a question, be prepared for the answer because the answer is also implicit in the question. Sometimes it is better not to ask. In New York, we used to say, 'Don't ask if you don't want to know'. Because once you ask, you will come to know. So when you ask, 'Who am I?' the answer is coming. If that becomes an important question to you, then your spiritual process is in high gear.

Every field of life is an inquiry. Philosophy asks, 'What is the meaning of life?' Science asks, 'How does this work? Why is this so?' Religion asks, 'What is God?' Darwinian evolution asks, 'Where did we come from?' Engineering asks, 'How can I get it to work?' All of the branches of human knowledge are structures built on questions. Such is the power of the question.

The inquiries I've mentioned are external and use the instrumentality of the mind. When the mind turns its inquiry power on itself, we have arrived at Self-inquiry, the last and certainly the most fundamental of all inquiries.

Inwardly, we continually ask ourselves questions. 'Should I marry this person? Should I take that job?' All through the day, our self-questioning goes on. 'Should I go to this program tonight?' or 'What should I watch on television?'

The flow of mundane questions continues. That we are always asking questions demonstrates our confidence that there is something or someone inside who is going to answer. You don't ask a stone a question (unless you're in India and it is painted orange, then you might).

THE INNER VOICE

Who, then, answers? Who gives you that answer? Here is one of the important issues that arises in Self-inquiry: we know that some answers are reliable and some answers are not reliable. You also doubtless know, looking back on choices you have made, that some of them were simply bad. Yes, I know everything happens for the best. But let's take off our New Age glasses for a moment. Look at some of your choices—that first husband or wife. It was very broadening, it helped your full development as a human being, no doubt, but in hindsight, it was a bad choice. At the time, you inquired: 'Should I do this or not?' Based on that inquiry, you did it. Later, you say, 'Oh, I always knew I shouldn't have done it!'

Doesn't that imply there were several voices, several opinions clamouring and you picked the wrong one? Now you feel that you always knew it was the wrong one. It is as though different parts of ourselves speak to us. Do you remember those cartoons when a character had a decision to make and a little devil is whispering into one ear and an angel into the other? The issue in Self-inquiry is to get in touch with the most true, the most real voice inside—the voice of the Self.

Lurking negative emotions distort the inner voice. If you are in an angry state and you consult your inner voice, you get an answer that is distorted by that anger. Didn't some wise older person tell you in your youth that if you are angry, you should not make any decisions? It's a pity if you didn't get that teaching. When you are angry, count to 10, or wait a day and calm down. That person probably told you to try to do everything from a balanced, calm space. Perhaps when you move from one kind of hysteria to another, you pass through calm for a moment, and that's when you should inquire.

If you are in a state of fear and paranoia and you ask yourself something, you get an answer distorted by that fear and paranoia. The same is true if you are under the sway of a strong desire. Under these conditions, your inner voice is not trustworthy. Gurdjieff says there are many I's within. Each emotion or mood creates a different 'I'. What is the seed of every thought and decision we make? When anger, fear or depression provides the seed, our decision-making and thinking capacity is compromised. Gurdjieff would say you are under the influence of a false 'I'. Another way to say this is that the answer you get is from the mind and not from the Self, or that your ego has kicked in.

In the first session of my Learn to Meditate course, I lead the Self-Inquiry Guided Chakra Meditation. (Play Track 1 or see Appendix E.) I ask the class to focus on the worst chakra, the one with the most tension, and then answer inwardly the following three questions.

What emotion is this feeling?

What caused this feeling? (The cause could be an encounter that happened today, or long ago; it could be an immediate issue or a chronic one, and so on.)

The third question, and perhaps the most important one, is 'What do I need to do to shift this feeling or ease this tension?' The answer might require an action in the outer world or a surrender or shift of understanding in the inner world. I tell my class not to create an answer with their mind and self-will, but let the inner Self answer.

I ask for a show of hands as to how many either received an answer to the third question or *maybe* received an answer. Ninety per cent of my students say they did. Who gives the answer? The wisdom of meditation tells us that when we attain clarity, our mind is most trustworthy. The voice of the Self issues from that space.

We have to learn to distinguish the multiple voices from the voice of the Self. This is an essential element of inquiry. Spiritually, inquiry aims at finding the voice of the Self. There are methods to find that voice, and it has identifiable characteristics.

THE TRADITION OF SELF-INQUIRY

The first time I heard about *atma vichara* was from the American spiritual teacher Ram Dass who was very much a part of my awakening back in 1970. He taught many techniques. He said, 'You should do some *pranayama*, some breath control. You should stare at a candle to calm the mind. You should burn incense before a picture of the deity. You should say a mantra'. And then he talked about Ramana Maharshi. All discussions of inquiry must begin with Sri Ramana. He is the godfather of inquiry. He is eternally joined to Self-inquiry. He is the one who developed it and popularised it in modern times.

Ramana's method begins with the question, 'Am I my body?' Seeing clearly that I am not my body, the inquirer asks, 'Am I my senses, am I my mind?' and so on, discovering that the Self is separate from anything that can be named or objectified. In Ram Dass' description, inquiry functions like an infinite regress that goes inward towards your centre, finally going through a doorway, where the inquirer becomes absorbed in the Self.

Intrigued, I went to a local bookstore and bought the book, *Talks with Sri Ramana Maharshi*, and I started to read it. Though I had trouble understanding much of it, it seemed like a deep ocean of wisdom.

Ramana's technique is sometimes called the 'Who am I?' meditation. You ask silently, 'Who am I?' Ramana was not the first who talked about inquiry. When I was in Ganeshpuri, we used to chant *Bhaja Govindam* or *Bhaja Gurudevam*, a chant written by Shankaracharya. There is a verse in it that says, 'Who are you? Who am I? Where have I come from? Who is my mother? Who is my father?' Shankaracharya used a questioning technique, 'Who am I? What is the purpose of my life? Where am I going?' Shankaracharya, remarkably, was using this kind of inquiry more than a thousand years ago.

Earlier even than Shankaracharya, there were veiled references to inquiry. In the *Katha Upanishad*, a young boy named Natchiketa has a dialogue with Lord Yama, the Prince of Death, and he is taught about the Self. Lord Yama teaches:

> The primeval one who is hard to perceive, wrapped in mystery, hidden in the cave of the heart, residing within the impenetrable depths: regarding him as God, an insight gained by inner contemplation, the wise abandon both sorrow and joy.

Here, the truth is 'wrapped in mystery, hidden in the cave', 'hard to perceive'. It is at an 'impenetrable depth'. This is inquiry: to penetrate the layers of ignorance, of illusion, and get to the kernel of light.

The *Bhagavad Gita* says:

> Little by little he should attain tranquillity by means of his firmly held intellect; he should establish the mind in the Self and abstain from every kind of thought.

In inquiry, the mind has to become steady. If the mind is unsteady, inquiry can't be done. There has to be focus, there has to be attention and there has to be silence—inner silence—to get to that place.

The interesting text, *Yoga Vashishta*, discusses inquiry in great detail, saying, among many other things, that it is a method for advanced seekers.

It is true that it is only possible for mature minds, not for immature ones. For the latter, repetition of a mantra under one's breath (*japa*), worship of images, breath-control (*pranayama*), visualising a pillar of light and similar yogic and spiritual and religious practices have been prescribed. By those practices, people become mature and will then realise the Self through the path of Self-inquiry.

Abhinavagupta concurs. He says:

Inquiry is the highest branch of yoga since it distinguishes between what is to be rejected and what is to be chosen. Therefore the wise person should practise inquiry.

As I have said, in the process of ordinary living we all practise an informal inquiry. Since we know how to do it informally, all we have to do is give it more rigour, and it will help us make wise and powerful choices in our lives. Abhinavagupta calls inquiry the 'wish-fulfilling cow which surpasses all other methods'. It is a 'finely sharpened axe, which cuts the root of the tree of duality'.

TRACK 4. INQUIRY: WHO AM I?

Ask inwardly, 'Who am I?' and become directly in touch with the context of all experience, which is your own Self. Say:

- I am awareness.

- I am the screen.

- I am the space.

- I am the feeling of Self.

Make these statements and reflect on each. These are in the spirit of Ramana's inquiry.

Alternatively, you can ask yourself, 'What is my awareness?' and get in touch with the place towards which that question points.

SOME MODERN YOGIS OF SELF-INQUIRY

'Who am I?' is not, for Ramana, a mantra to be repeated, and it is also not a question to be answered mentally. Nonetheless, there are yogis who have taught it in both of these ways. One used the method of two people sitting opposite each other. One asks the other, 'Who are you?' Whatever answer is received, they again ask, 'Who are you?' And again and again. The idea is that this process takes them to deeper layers of reality. Osho, a popular Indian Guru of the '70s and '80s, had a wild technique in which people would dance and call out, 'Who? Who? Who?' But these are not Ramana's methods. He used 'Who am I?' to return the mind to a clean slate. Ramana's method is designed to chop off the story and the drama, to return to the clear space of Consciousness.

A contemporary yogi, Da Avabhasa, developed a kind of inquiry based on the question 'Avoiding relationship?' Its rationale is something like this: the universe is one. The reality of the universe is that there is oneness. There is one Consciousness everywhere, but we don't always experience oneness. We experience duality, we experience separation. We experience tension and contraction. When that tension arises, we should inquire inwardly, 'Avoiding relationship?' Since you are a part of a whole that has suddenly become separate, you must be doing something to avoid your natural state of relationship with the whole. Are you fighting the river or being part of the flow? With that inquiry, you bring yourself back into relationship.

> ### INQUIRY: AVOIDING RELATIONSHIP?
>
> Go inside and look for places of tension. You may notice a block in one or a number of areas. If you feel one, ask into it, 'Avoiding relationship?' and see what arises.

SRI RAMANA'S SELF-INQUIRY

Let's go on now to consider Ramana's method. Ramana wrote an interesting little text called *Who Am I?* in which he describes his technique of inquiry. In my early *sadhana*, I tried to understand his method. I read and reread his works but something still eluded me. After arriving at the ashram in Ganeshpuri, I put Ramana's book away and spent six months doing the demanding *sadhana* there. When I picked up the book again, to my amazement, it made perfect sense and seemed completely lucid to me.

That was an important moment. I had undergone a variety of experiences, but I had no idea if I was progressing. When you are in the maelstrom of *sadhana*, you lose sight of the big picture. When I read Ramana's book with new comprehension, I saw that something fundamental had changed dramatically. It confirmed that my *sadhana* was going well.

Ramana says:

> Therefore, making the corpse-body remain as a corpse, and not even uttering the word 'I', one should inquire keenly thus: 'Now, what is it that rises as "I"?'

This is meaningful in the context of Ramana's own story. Ramana had one of the most extraordinary *sadhanas* ever recorded. It was completed in less than half an hour. He was a 16-year-old boy from South India, with no particular spirituality in his background. One afternoon he was in his uncle's apartment by himself and was suddenly gripped by a fear of death. He lay down on the floor and asked himself, 'If my body dies, will I die?'

This arose spontaneously. He saw that *he* would still be alive, even if the body died. 'Well then, who am I? Am I my mind? If my mind goes, will I go?' You should understand that this was no wordy intellectual process. He was in a state of tension and fear. His inquiry was fuelled by the emotion that gripped him. In 20 minutes, he realised the Self. He had done no practice before that. Let me emphasise that. Every spiritual seeker who comes across Ramana's astonishing account turns green with envy. He must have done his yoga in past lives and had very little left to do. After that experience, he was permanently established in the Self.

In Indian music, the shruti is a drone-like sound provided by a tamboura or a squeezebox. It functions like the bass line in the West—

it creates a steady context. Ramana said that after his experience, the Self was with him like the drone of the *shruti*. It became the background music that was always there.

After realisation, he had no interest in school or anything mundane, and he would sit on his bed with his schoolbooks open, falling into meditation. Noticing this, his brother said to him sarcastically, 'Hey, if you are such a *sadhu* (holy being), why don't you leave home and go to the Himalayas?' And Ramana thought, 'Good idea!' Soon after that, he was gone, leaving a note for his parents. He went to the holy mountain Arunachala, in South India, where he spent the rest of his life.

Arunachala served as a kind of Guru to him and, once there, he fell into a deep state of *samadhi* (meditative trance) that lasted many months. His state was such that he didn't feed himself, he was filthy, his hair grew, his nails grew, and he was covered with insects that bit him. Here in the West, I don't know what we would do with such a person. But in India they recognised that he was a holy man, and they valued him and took care of him. After about a year, he came out of his intense absorption and started to talk to people. They asked him spiritual questions and, having no knowledge of the scriptures, he answered solely from his own direct experience. To help the devotees, he studied the scriptures himself in order to answer their questions. His reaction to the scriptures was, 'Oh yes, they're correct. They're quite right'.

It is said that the sages teach the path they themselves walked. If someone asks you how to get to Mt Eliza, you will probably tell them the way you came. There are two highways that come here, but generally you will teach the way you came yourself. Ramana's whole *sadhana* and the seeds of everything he taught later were all in that half-hour of his realisation. The method of inquiry he has made so famous arose then.

In *Self-Inquiry*, Ramana tells us to regard the body as a corpse and then inquire keenly: 'Now, what is it that arises as "I"?' The meditator leaves the body for dead, reflecting Ramana's original experience, then searches for the Self within, 'What is the "I"? Who am I?' Now he moves beyond the words 'Who am I?' to a feeling in the heart. Ramana calls it 'a kind of wordless illumination of the form "I-I"'. Krishnamurti called the same place 'choiceless awareness'. Ramana refers not to the words 'I-I', but to the flow of I-Consciousness. If, in this practice, a thought arises, the inquirer is to ask within, 'To whom does this thought belong? Who is thinking this thought?' That takes him back to the flow of I-awareness.

If you say 'I am' or 'I', you are still in the realm of language. Prior to the word is the feeling of 'I'. Ramana points us to this feeling sense of 'I' in the heart, a kind of shining in the heart. His inquiry goes from the body to the mind, to the word and beyond the word to the actual direct experience or feeling-experience of the 'I'. That is what he is talking about. That is his whole *sadhana*. You simply hold on to the feeling sense of 'I'.

The thought 'I am' is the first thought as Consciousness comes into manifestation, and the last thought as manifestation merges in Consciousness. It is thus the doorway to the Self. The meditator can get to the 'I am' thought by an inner movement of will. To go beyond that, however, grace is necessary. Thus, in the path of wisdom, the inquirer is sometimes asked to find the 'I am' and sit in it, by a subtle inner effort.

INQUIRY: I AM

In Ramana's *atma vichara*, he tells us the Self is in the cave of the heart. Take the words, 'I am' and use that 'I am' as a pointer to direct you into the heart where your sense of Self is. Let go of the words 'I am' and be with the feeling of Self. Notice where in the body the 'I am' shows up (there is no single correct answer for this). Be with the 'I am' for as long as you can. Try to relax into it and let Consciousness take you. Nothing metaphysical, intellectual or complex, just your own ordinary sense of Self.

Alternatively, you can ask the 'I am' what it has to tell you, either spiritually or regarding concrete issues.

Shaivism says the I-sense is *fundamental* to Consciousness. It should not be eliminated; indeed, it cannot be eliminated. The I-sense is Consciousness' experience of interiority. *Only* Consciousness has the sense of intimacy or interiority. Some schools of thought hold that the I-sense is eliminated as Consciousness is purified. But interiority is nothing but love, and it is intrinsic to Consciousness.

The problem is not the existence of the sense of 'I', but that we associate it with our personhood, our body-mind, when it actually belongs to Shiva. The normal, habitual, friendly 'I' that each of us feels is, in fact, the supreme I-Consciousness at the core of our reality. Thus, if we ride our normal sense of self inward, we arrive at our identity with the supreme person; Shiva. Ramana's teaching is in harmony with this point of view. Inquiry into the I-power of awareness leads directly to the perspective of impersonal Consciousness, and shows the relationship between the personal and the impersonal.

THE EGO AND THE WITNESS

Ramana finds the seeds of our spiritual bondage in the ego, which arises as the first thought that comes from the I-sense. The ego is the expression of the misidentification of the Self with the body, thus the first thought of the ego is 'I am the body'. All other thoughts are based on this original mistake. Chop down the ego and you uproot the tree of ignorance; the proliferation of mental structures that constitutes our bondage.

When there is a problem, we have to go to the seed, the source of the problem. Once the seed is destroyed, the problem ceases to exist. In this case, however, Ramana sets us no small task. We have to discard our entire mental and emotional life.

> Whatever thoughts arise as obstacles to one's *sadhana*, the mind should not be allowed to go in their direction, but should be made to rest in one's Self.

When you focus on the heart, you will notice that thoughts continue to arise. Here, the task of the meditator is to hold the mind in the Self, and resist the temptation to let the mind's thoughts do the leading.

In the technique of witness-consciousness, you observe the thoughts and let them come and go. You don't fight them off or try to repress them, but you don't run off with them either. Ramana suggests the attitude, 'Let whatever strange things happen, happen. Let us see'. This should be one's practice. One should not identify oneself with appearances; one should never relinquish one's Self.

CONTEMPLATION: WITNESS-CONSCIOUSNESS

Hold the Self, and then have the attitude, 'Let's see what is going to happen. Unexpected things are going to come up, let's see what they are'. Have a little excitement, a little interest. 'Let whatever strange things happen, happen.' Very funny about the mind—you never know what it's going to produce, do you? It's quite amazing this mind, this thought-factory. Witnessing the thoughts in this way leads to mastery of the mind.

GIVING BODY TO INQUIRY

For Ramana, thinking itself is bondage: 'The best discipline is to stay quiescent without ever forgetting the Self.' Ramana's practice is uncompromising. Thought is bondage. He says, 'Don't think. Don't think. Don't think!'

There is truth in the doctrine of 'no thought' but it is also misleading. It conjures the image of an enlightened master who is like other people in every way except that he or she has no mind. Where others have their thinking apparatus in place, an inner voice that chatters endlessly, one imagines that a realised sage has an empty space. But realisation is not about killing the mind in that sense.

Bad actions that you perform with your hands and arms can bind you, but you don't have to chop your arms off to be Self-realised. You simply cease to misuse your organs of action. In the same way, you don't have to kill the mind, but, rather, stop misusing it. Thought is natural for a human being. But there are thoughts that bind you and thoughts that don't. When a thought is full of negative emotion or delusion and contracts you, then it binds you. But if thoughts occur without a negative and contracting effect, then they don't bind you.

This is where our method of Self-inquiry comes in. The mind-free practice that Ramana suggests is based on stillness, pure stillness—going beyond the mind. This is Shaivite *shambhavopaya*. It is an exalted path and a valid one. However, language defines human life. What do we do that isn't connected to language? Apart from deep sleep, everything is about language. The defining characteristic of a human being is language. What separates man from the animal is language ability.

According to Shaivism, Self-realisation has two aspects that relate to the inner world and outer world respectively. The first, *atma vyapti* (immersion in the Self) implies the stillness of deep meditation. Here, meditators do indeed silence their minds in the Self and attain *nirvikalpa samadhi*, deep conscious trance.

But this attainment, significant as it is, does not bring full realisation. There must also be the second, *Shiva vyapti*, immersion in universal Consciousness. Here, meditators bring their *samadhi* state into their outer life. With eyes open, they live with complete peace and unity Consciousness.

In this state, also traditionally called *sahaja samadhi*, natural liberation, their minds do exist as a major player in their life and life choices. The Shaivite sage Utpaladeva says, loosely translated, that in this state a yogi is liberated 'even though thoughts play in his mind'. For such yogis, the mind is their servant and their tool, not their master. It is not at the service of negative emotions or haphazard thoughts, but is the servant only of the Self.

The *Yoga Vashishta* says:

> The eye of spiritual inquiry does not lose its sight even in the midst of all activities; he who does not have this eye is indeed to be pitied ... Knowledge of truth arises from such inquiry; from such knowledge there follows tranquillity in oneself; and then arises supreme peace ... and the ending of all sorrow.

I think it is essential to bring Self-inquiry down to earth and give it a body, and also a mind and a tongue. It needs to come into the real world. There is not only *atma vyapti* but also *Shiva vyapti*. There is not only the method of *shambhavopaya*, there is also *shaktopaya*—the way of the mind—and *anavopaya*—the way of the body. Ramana, as great as he was, has spawned legions of immature *jnanis*—people who want to bypass the mind and body, and rocket directly to the Self. It is doubtful that it can be done. You have to work *with* the mind. You have to purify the mind. If you try to skip over the mind, you may briefly attain *samadhi*, but you will still have an impure mind. And it will continue to give you trouble when you come out of *samadhi*.

Remember that Ramana realised the Self easily. Moreover, his personality was austere and detached. He had little vital energy. He was a sage who was content to stay in retreat for his whole life. As a consequence, his method is rarefied. It is suitable for highly qualified seekers in a monastic context. On the other hand, inquiry can be tremendously valuable for everyone, not only at the highest spiritual level—the *shambhavopaya* level—but at the level of practical life. You can bring it into your body. It can help you with physical problems. It can help you in your career. It can help you in your relationships. The Shiva Process is Shaivite inquiry. It brings the disembodied Vedantic inquiry down into living situations. It gives us a spiritual tool for understanding everything in our physical, mental and emotional worlds. And, of course, it can be used on the highest spiritual level as well.

THE CLEAR SPACE OF GOOD FEELING

When I went to India seeking enlightenment, having come out of the '60s, I thought of enlightenment as a kind of psychedelic state. An abiding contact with the Self is extraordinary in many ways, but these days I prefer to speak about enlightenment in more ordinary terms. We don't need to grow new faculties; our ordinary human faculties, *properly handled*, are sufficient. If we could see, hear, think and feel in the way that the instruments of these actions were designed to function, we would have enlightenment. We would be able to perceive things as they are. Our minds would operate with clarity and intelligence, our emotions would stay in the zone of peacefulness and love, and our actions would be appropriate and compassionate.

Because the inner world consists of a thought element and an emotional element, I acknowledge both of these in my formulation, the clear space of good feeling. The intellectual faculties are clear: the feeling is good. In such a state, a person is both wise and loving. This state is our natural condition, and we practise inquiry to remove the disturbing elements that obscure it. People sometimes ask me how long their spiritual work has to go on; that it seems unending. I say that every time the clear space of good feeling is lost, it has to be recovered. If you don't lose that space, you don't have to seek it. It's not the path that is endless, but our bad habits can seem endless.

Actions that flow from a clear space of good feeling are effective actions. Actions that flow from another inner space are distorted to the extent that the generating space differs from the clear space of good feeling. Therefore, a yogi of inquiry should always be aware of the underlying seed, the space that sources their words and actions. When that space is not the clear space of good feeling, Self-inquiry must be pursued to recover it.

An intelligent person tries to keep the clear space of good feeling at all times. When bad feeling enters, a yogi tries to move it, to clear it through A-, B- and G-Statements, taking action, praying and so on. Ego and attachment take you out of that clear space, whereas right understanding keeps you in it. An enlightened sage is one who remains in that clear space of good feeling. In group-inquiry, the group, too, tries to attain and maintain that clear space.

INQUIRY:
FINDING THE CLEAR SPACE OF GOOD FEELING

Turn within and find the clear space of good feeling. Have the faith that it is somewhere there inside you. Once you attain the clear space of good feeling, listen to the voice of the Self. Ask inwardly what it has to tell you.

FOLLOW YOUR BEST IDEA

Self-inquiry develops right understanding, which the Buddha calls right view. Let's say you are playing a game of rugby but you think you're playing American football. The games are close enough to each other that even with your 'wrong view', you'll occasionally get things right and do something good. The rest of the time, things won't work out as well for reasons you won't be able to understand. So, right understanding means to understand how the game is set up, what the rules are and what the goal is. It's quite astounding that most of us don't have a clue about any of these basic things.

I recently saw a movie in which the characters were in a bad situation and mulling over alternatives. One of them said, 'You have to follow your best idea' and I had a flash of revelation. Isn't everyone always following their best idea? Of course they are. And isn't it funny or sad that our best idea is so often inadequate? That's the game of life: following your best idea. If we want to follow our best idea, why is it we come up with such bad ideas? Here is where inquiry comes in. Bad ideas come from *raga/dvesha*, attachment and aversion. Because of our wants and fears, we don't have enough detachment to establish right view and know what to do. Inquiry can penetrate the confusion of attachment and aversion, and bring us to at least a better, if not the best, idea that we can hold.

MATRIKA: PURIFYING THE MIND

A significant aphorism in Shaivism says, *Jnanadhishthanam matrika*: 'The letters of the alphabet are the source of all knowledge.' Language creates our universe. Language brings us up, language brings us down, language expands us, and language contracts us. The words we say to others have an uplifting effect or a contracting effect. The words we speak as thoughts inside our own brain similarly expand us or contract us. It is not enough just to go into the silence. We have to become aware of the self-talk, the *matrika*, that goes on inside. We have to see it clearly and comprehensively. We can't leave any part of it out. We have to balance ourselves on every level of our being.

Not that Ramana didn't know that; of course he did. His dialogues reveal that a lot of his teaching was practical and less absolutist. He did tell people to go beyond the mind, but he also told them to work with the mind and purify it of negative emotions, desire and inertia.

When you read an Indian text, you will notice many references to the mind, but you will probably look in vain for a discussion of the emotions. In the West, we are enormously interested in the emotions. When the Indian yogis refer to the 'mind', they mean both thought and feeling. They simply don't distinguish them as we do. The yogic texts say that the mind is sometimes coloured by *rajas* and *tamas*, the qualities of desire and ignorance. Such a mind holds negative emotions—anger, fear, despair and similar negative qualities. When the mind is under their influence, it cannot know the Self.

The mind has to be gradually purified and refined. That involves getting rid of negative emotions, getting rid of depression, getting rid of fear, anger and anxiety. It has to become more peaceful. Does it mean that it will never be afflicted by wrong movements? Not necessarily. The mind is a plastic medium and receptive to all kinds of thoughts. However, the mind of a *jnani* is capable of getting rid of negative emotions by the application of wisdom power. All the great beings have done this.

As I've said, Ramana's path to realisation was short and easy. But many realised beings had to do it the old-fashioned way, through a long spiritual ordeal and painful self-mastery. My own Guru did it the hard way. Even after meeting his Guru, he did nine more years of hard work. When I met Baba, he was an extraordinary being, but he had been an ordinary person earlier in his life. Then, through effort, strong intention and dedication to the path, he broke through and achieved the goal.

Ramana aside, the spiritual process requires patience and steady and gradual practice. Over an extended period of earnest practice, the mind, almost invisibly, comes to work more positively. The frequency of negative thoughts is decreased and the frequency of positive thoughts is increased. Just as a child grows imperceptibly, but then one day is six feet tall, so the mind's transformation is invisible. Then suddenly a situation arises in which our behaviour is clearly more controlled and conscious than it has been in the past.

Or we have a sudden glimpse of ourselves as a whole and see clearly that a global change has happened. As inquiry continues, the mind becomes more subtle and more expanded. It now becomes capable of grasping the truth. Such a mind has become ripe for knowledge of the Self.

> ### INQUIRY: WHO IS THINKING THIS THOUGHT?
>
> Go within and ask yourself, 'Who am I?' You can answer in any superficial way you want: your social role, your physical identity and your political or religious beliefs. Search for deeper answers. Finally, get yourself to the feeling of 'I am'. Let go of the *thought* 'I am', and experience the *feeling* of it—the wordless, thoughtless state of Self-awareness. When other thoughts come in, reject them the way Ramana would, by saying, 'Who is thinking this thought?' Hold the feeling experience of the Self. Do this inquiry for as long as you can, without straining. Then, meditate normally.

QUESTIONS AND ANSWERS

TRUSTING THE INNER VOICE

Question: It seems to me that I have trust issues and that even if I heard the voice of the Self, I wouldn't believe it. Do you have any suggestions?

Swamiji: It's not so much that you have trust issues as you have doubt issues. You have a habit of doubting everything and you need to see it and overcome it. The kind of trust I'm talking about is not the kind of trust we associate with blind faith. In that kind of trust, somebody says, 'Trust me, it's this way'; you say, 'I don't feel good about it'.

What I'm talking about is trusting and going with the sense of harmony and peace that certain choices give you. If the Self tells you this is correct, trust that feeling or intuition. Then a voice arises and wonders if it's wrong. That is just your habit of doubt. Get rid of it. Trusting the good inner feeling can lead you into unexpected territory. It can stretch you and help you grow.

Paying attention to the voice of the Self, the upward shift of feeling, actually entails a new way of living, a new criterion of choice. It is a criterion beyond the mind. Here's something you can trust: the Self is stronger than the mind. It might look as though your mind completely defeats you at every turn, but in fact it's far too weak, flighty, indulgent, negative (add whatever adjective you like). Despite appearances, it's an unequal struggle that the Self will win. I've been doing this for a long time and I don't doubt this; I have seen so much improvement in so many people and dozens of extraordinary transformations.

THOUGHT AND FEELING

Question: Could you talk a little more about thought and feeling?

Swamiji: Whenever anyone asks me this, and they do, the thought leaps into my mind, 'Two sides of the same coin!' You can't really separate thought and feeling. Good feeling always goes with positive thinking and bad feeling always goes with negative thinking. Thought is form because it shapes reality, while feeling is essence. When the form we create is a negative thought, the feeling that it creates is negative. I like the analogy of a balloon. When the balloon is in its natural condition, the air in it is positive and exuberant. When you twist and squeeze the balloon (negative thinking), it increases in tension and screeches (negative feeling). So we have to shape the thinking side of the equation properly and then the essence, the feeling, will happily reflect it.

RAMANA AND VEDANTA

Question: Is Ramana's 'Who am I?' inquiry the same as Vedanta's *Neti, neti*: 'Not this, not this?'

Swamiji: When all is said and done, they are similar. 'Who am I?' is very much in the Vedantic spirit of eliminating our identification: 'I'm not this, I'm not that.' Where Vedanta rejects, Shaivism embraces. When I say the Shaivite point of view, 'Everything is Consciousness', I am saying, 'I am everything. I am my body'. But I am not *in* my body. My body is in *me*. Your body is in you. You are not in your body. Can you understand that perspective? If your *awareness* is who you are, then your body is just one thing in your awareness. Shaivism says we are all of this.

SCIENCE AND RELIGION

Question: One of the things I like about your method of Self-inquiry is it doesn't seem to be a religious activity. Could you comment on that?

Swamiji: Yes, I agree with you. Although you'd have to admit that it is spiritual, which is religion in its highest form. I sometimes think of Self-inquiry as inner-world science. Science is objective, analytical and experimental, but neglects the world of feeling and the possibility of a higher power. Religion, on the other hand, has feeling and intuition, but it can also have dogma and arbitrary rules and tradition. Self-inquiry is where science meets religion, without dogma, but with feeling; without the coldness of science, but with its objective experimental approach.

It is 'objective subjectivity'. You look at your inner world with the cool vision of a scientist, with no expectations or preconceptions, to discover what is there. You are both the scientist and the experiment. Your goal is to discover what *is* and to also find a working technology of positive transformation. The spiritual teacher Douglas Harding would call it first-person science, as opposed to outer-world science, which is third-person science.

Perhaps the most extraordinary feature of Consciousness is that it has interiority. To know something from within is always different from knowing something from without. And it is not an invalid way of knowing something. On the contrary, I would call it the most valid of all ways of knowing.

Question: Are science and religion forever opposed?

Swamiji: Science and religion are like two people approaching the same stream from opposite banks. They want to merge in the same water, but they don't know it, just as psychology really wants to become yoga, but doesn't know it. Science has objective thought and experimental method. Both of these are powerful tools and yield results. But the downside of science is that it neglects the subjective and emotional side. It is without any notion of a higher power. It is dry in these ways.

On the other hand, while religion has a notion of a higher power, its thinking function is less precise and free than that of science. Religious thought can be dogmatic; it lacks science's free, experimental method. Science has the virtue, at least in principle, of being free-spirited in its inquiry.

One of the key things about science is that its experiments and its findings are repeatable. Science would be useless if an experiment that I conduct can't be repeated by somebody else in a different time and place. Each time you do the experiment and get the same results, you strengthen the evidence in favour of your hypothesis. In this way, Self-inquiry is scientific and empirical. Dogmatic religion involves accepting things that some authority professes, but Self-inquiry is an ongoing experiment and the results should be repeatable. This is a useful attitude for the practitioner of Shiva Process to hold: the result I get today is evidence but the process may have to be repeated to be certain.

When science finally surrenders its quixotic quest to eliminate the observer—the subject—it will have no choice but to move towards that subject and inquire into it. It is well known that 20th-century physics has acknowledged that the presence of an observer (that is, the scientist) changes the situation and the experiment. According to Utpaladeva, whatever is known must be known by some knower, therefore objectivity is a myth dreamt up by some highly imaginative subject. Dreamers dream of a world in which they do not exist. They can never know that world, because if they did, they would have to be there.

INQUIRY IN THE WEST

Question: In your opinion, is Self-inquiry completely absent from Western thought?

Swamiji: No, it isn't, although I think it was not brought to perfection. A well-known form of philosophical inquiry in the West is Socratic inquiry. If you read Plato's dialogues, Socrates is always questioning, deconstructing the opinions and ideas of whomever he's speaking to. He takes the stance that he knows nothing; that he is merely a 'midwife' who helps the other person give birth to what they really believe. But by the end of each dialogue, you are convinced the person he is speaking to surely knows nothing.

The most impressive and important bit of philosophical inquiry in the West is undoubtedly that of René Descartes. As a solitary inner voyager with no supporting spiritual tradition, his achievement is impressive. Even though he fell short of the goal of real inquiry, I would give him an A+. Descartes' investigation was a search for what he knew for certain. As he inquired, he discovered that most of what he thought he knew was actually hearsay and indirect knowledge; 'mere opinion'.

He even felt his senses might be lying to him. Finally, he made his famous statement, *Cogito ergo sum*: 'I think therefore I am.' A yogi knows that Descartes was one step short of grabbing the brass ring. A yogi might say, 'I am and I also think'. In other words, Descartes equates the self with the thinking mind and doesn't arrive at the intuition of the Self as the witness of the mind or pure Consciousness. Nonetheless, bravo René; great work for a lone explorer. Descartes' inquiry had such a powerful impact on Western thought that even today, centuries later, his findings are still hotly debated by scientists and philosophers in the field of Consciousness.

I'm quite sure that in the spiritual realm, forms of inquiry were developed by Christian contemplatives. For example, you might look at the work of Saint Ignatius of Loyola, compiler of *Spiritual Exercises*, a set of considerations, prayers, thought experiments and examinations of Consciousness. I'm aware of the work of the Hasid, Rebbe Nachman of Breslav, who created a unique form of inner dialogue, which borders on inquiry. It's true that Western inquiry, while it was exceptionally strong, was generally directed at outer objects. It manifested powerfully as science and technology. Once that same skill is turned to the inner world, Western Self-inquiry will flourish.

THREE GOALS OF SELF-INQUIRY

Question: What are the goals of Self-inquiry?

Swamiji: The goal is to attain the Self. As I've mentioned, I like to define that in more practical terms as the clear space of good feeling. Clear space implies mental clarity. Good feeling hints at emotional peace and positivity. Thus, clarity, peace and joy are the goals.

Once we find the clear space of good feeling, a fourth goal becomes possible, and that is right action. Good actions emerge from a clear space of good feeling, while bad or wrong actions emerge from the 'confused space of bad feeling'. The Shiva Process always wants you to put your understandings into appropriate action in your life.

The aim is to banish anyone who has invaded your inner space. Get rid of everyone but the Self. That includes your ego, your persona and anyone else who has crept in!

SEEKING THE SHADOW

Question: I find that I have strong opinions on different things: political opinions, personal opinions, religious opinions. I notice that I get burned when I express them too forcibly. Could you comment on this?

Swamiji: You know, ardent atheists, when they get religion, become religious fanatics. Isn't that almost a cliché? In your life, there must surely be one or two areas in which your beliefs now are 180 degrees different from your beliefs in the past.

Since Shiva contains all opposites, taking passionate positions separates us from Him. A passionate position defines us and limits us. Still, we are human beings and human beings should have passionate opinions. But while having your opinions in your human way, remember that, given a different context, you might believe the opposite. I think there is a shadow person within each of us who holds totally different opinions, especially where we're most passionate. We have put that shadow person into our unconscious and we have a war with them. We may have to become that person in a future life.

You should find your shadow person in meditation and harmonise them with your present opinionated person. Then go beyond both to the divine person who contains them both. In meditation, you can actively cancel your opinions: your political ideas, your spiritual ideas and your moral ideas. This won't have a bad effect on you. You will still hold your opinions, but in a less attached way, knowing they are not eternal truths. If you make peace now with your shadow person and bring them out of the shadows, you will not have to be reborn as that person, casting your present identity into the shadows.

SUMMARY

- Inquiry makes us aware of our moment-to-moment reactions.

- A question is a technique by which Consciousness is focused.

- A question is not far from its answer.

- The goal in Self-inquiry is to get in touch with the most true inner voice; the voice of the Self.

- Ramana's inquiry features the question 'Who am I?'

- Ramana's inquiry goes beyond language and thought to the feeling sense of 'I' in the heart.

- Ego is misidentification with the body.

- Self-inquiry is a means to return to a clear space of good feeling.

- It is important to work with the mind's self-talk to purify it.

- Self-inquiry can be used in every aspect of life.

- Good feeling goes with positive thinking and bad feeling goes with negative thinking.

- Self-inquiry applies scientific method to the inner world.

- Self-inquiry is where science meets religion without dogma.

- The goal of Self-inquiry is to attain the Self.

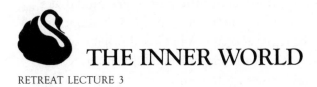

THE INNER WORLD

Life and all else are in Brahman alone.
Brahman is here and now. Investigate.
Sri Ramana Maharshi

Bring your Self into focus, become aware of your own existence.
See how you function, watch the motives and the results
of your actions. Study the prison you have built
around yourself, by inadvertence.
Sri Nisargadatta Maharaj

There in he goes on worshipping whole heartedly the great
God, Lord Shiva, known as the supreme Bhairava,
along with his divine power Shakti with the
pure offerings of self-contemplation.
Abhinavagupta

THE MIND HAS the capacity to create confusion. In fact, confusion belongs entirely to the mind and to nowhere else. Self-inquiry gives us an effective alternative. While the mind says, 'think these thoughts, follow these mental possibilities', inquiry says, 'be present, investigate present experience'. In every moment, a choice can be made: do we follow the mind or do we stay with present experience?

I always feel a little guilty discoursing intellectually on something as experiential as inquiry. Therefore, to assuage my guilt, I will begin this lecture with a contemplation that highlights awareness of present experience.

TRACK 5. CONTEMPLATION: BECOMING PRESENT

Close your eyes, think about the past; everything that's happened leading to this moment has gone. Think about the future; the future has not yet come. What's real, what's actual, is the present moment. In the present moment, listen to the sounds. Now feel the sensations in your body—the sensation of sitting, your neck, your back. Now be aware of your breath coming in, going out. You've breathed a lot in the past, you will breathe in the future; the only breath that gives you air is the present breath. Breathe that breath.

Now turning to the inner world, become aware of your mind, of thoughts in your mind. The mind is thinking. We're not concerned with the content of the thoughts, but just that thoughts are occurring. Be aware of thoughts. At the same time, there's a feeling aspect of your inner experience. Be aware of your feeling or your mood in present time. It doesn't matter what the mood is, just be aware that there is some feeling, some mood.

Going deeper, go to the sense of 'I'. Say 'I am' and feel the feeling of being you in this moment. The feeling sense of 'I'—it's the most intimate, most personal, closest to the centre feeling: 'I am.'

Now we're present and I can go back to the past to the extent of a little summary of Lecture 2. I spoke about Sri Ramana Maharshi, whose method is to contemplate 'Who am I?' ever more subtly. As you do this contemplation, you say, 'I am not the body. I am not the mind' and so on, until you cannot go any further. Ultimately, your only identification is with Consciousness itself.

Ramana says:

> Make the mind take the form of the Self. In the middle of the heart-cave, the pure awareness is directly manifest as the Self in the form of 'I-I'.

'I-I' is his code for the feeling of Self. If you trace where your actual identity is, the feeling of 'I', you can find it in the heart; in the 'heart-cave'.

Take the mind and hold it in the Self. Don't let it rise up into thought. It wants to go up into the head and think. But if you trace it subtly, you find that the source of the mind is in the heart. This is what Ramana said.

The Self-inquiry we do here at the ashram expands Ramana's area of concern. While Ramana always points exclusively to the highest spiritual truth, our form of inquiry can be applied to everything in life.

I have already emphasised that we live in two worlds, the outer world and the inner world. And there are precisely two sorts of things in our inner world: *thought* and *feeling*. Thought and feeling, it turns out, are closely related—intimately related. It may not be intuitively obvious, but on investigation we see they are inextricably linked. When thought is positive, feeling is positive. When thought is negative, feeling is negative. You can test this for yourself in your own experience.

You can take it as a given that if you feel depressed, there must be *tearing thoughts* going on, whether you see them or not. Tearing thoughts are negative thoughts, especially those which tear into the thinker, like 'I am a loser' or 'I am worthless'. They attack the heart and undermine self-esteem.

If you are depressed, then tearing thoughts are in the neighbourhood. Given that clue, you can find them, because once you look for them, you will discover what is really going on inwardly.

Our feeling state, in any moment, is the result of the story we are telling ourselves within our own heads. Today, somebody said to me, 'I'm telling myself things that make me sad'. That is a useful way to articulate it. If you are angry, you could say, 'I am telling myself things that make me angry'. That gives a different perspective, doesn't it? The story you tell yourself about whatever happens creates your reaction.

The way we meet events in the moment we experience them determines everything: we get angry, we get depressed, we feel good. And that all has to do with the script we have inside. Two people have the same external experience, but they have a totally different emotional experience. Different scripts are working.

THE THREE TYPES: THINKING, FEELING, DOING

If you have been doing spiritual practice for a while, you have undoubtedly encountered a number of typologies that categorise and define personality types. Astrology is one such typology, the Enneagram is another, and Carl Jung created another. My favourite, which I like for its elegant simplicity, is also probably the most ancient, going back to the theory of the three *gunas*, constituents of the material universe, in the Sanskrit texts. Gurdjieff developed these insights, describing three aspects of a person: the intellectual aspect, the emotional aspect and the doing aspect.

Earlier, I mentioned that, depending on which one is more prominent, an individual belongs to the intellectual type, the emotional type or the doing type. In recent years, Da Avabhasa gave these types the colourful names, *Solid* (intellectual), *Peculiar* (emotional) and *Vital* (doing).

Each type relates to the outer world differently and they relate to their own inner worlds differently as well. Intellectual types pay more attention to the thought content of their inner world. They always notice the thought process, but may not be aware of the emotional process that occurs simultaneously. If you believe that you have small and unimportant feelings, but your thoughts are significant, you are probably a Solid. The data you select defines your world. My hatha yoga teacher in India, Baba Hari Dass, used to say that to a pickpocket, the world is nothing but pockets. Other people don't notice pockets. Your world reflects your interest.

While the thinking type pays attention to thought, the emotional type pays attention to feeling. If you hold the belief, 'My feelings are very big', I'd wager that you are a Peculiar. These are just clues. Everything is held in the attitude. There are people who tell me, 'I have this *huge* feeling! *Huge!*' Such people might profit by the contemplation, 'My feelings are smaller'.

For the doing type, whatever data they get inside spurs them to action. If a thought arises, they want to act on it. If a feeling arises, they want to act on it. Whatever happens inside, it's, 'Let's do something about it!' Vitals think a little, feel a little, but mostly act, like a rock crashing down a mountain. Vitals I have known have been superb at 'getting things done', but sometimes they do the wrong thing at the wrong time. Meditation tempers the vital impulse with wisdom and awareness.

Hold this typology lightly and it will give you insights. A surprisingly large number of people can't distinguish thought from feeling or feeling from sensation. As inquiry goes on, these important distinctions become clarified. By introspection, we can relatively easily distinguish a thought, which is characterised by language and ideas, and is associated with the mind. It's a little harder to differentiate a feeling from a sensation. Both feelings and sensations are non-verbal. A feeling is related to emotion and a sensation has to do with a physical response to the environment.

What is the characteristic of being thought-oriented? Thought gives strength and consistency; you are a person of principle and that makes you reliable. Feeling is not like that. Feeling goes up and down and you adopt different thoughts at different stages of the wave— completely different thoughts. You have an entirely different thought process when you are happy compared with when you are angry.

For people who are thought-oriented, it doesn't matter what feelings they have, their thought remains the same. The feeling person has, by compensation, an abundance of compassion and sympathy.

People who have strong principles live those principles. They are willing to sacrifice for those principles and even give up their lives for them. Through inquiry, we become aware of both sides of the ledger—thought and feeling. We are likely to be deficient in one or the other. We have to marry thought and feeling and bring them into balance.

When thought goes off on its own without reference to feeling, intellect loses touch with human compassion and sympathy. If you go in the other direction—just feeling—your life has no form, no intentionality. It simply goes up and down according to the winds of chance. Someone says something negative to you or a tearing thought comes in and you become deflated. Someone says something nice to you and you become inflated. In this way, you go up and down with events, without a stable centre.

TRUTH AND KINDNESS

Earlier, I mentioned the polarity of truth and kindness; that the place of empowerment is the place where truth is in balance with kindness. In our inquiry, we look for that balance point. Thought is truth, and feeling is kindness. Kindness without any truth doesn't have much strength. On the other hand, if you have all truth without any kindness or compassion, then you might go off in an inhuman, lunatic direction. We need to have both truth and kindness.

Real truth is also compassionate. It is not the 'harsh truth' or the 'hard truth'. Sometimes, trying to be kind, we repress the truth and don't stand up for ourselves. We don't want to say anything to upset anybody, yet because of that we lose energy. But where energy exists, where Shakti exists, where wisdom exists, is exactly the point where truth and kindness meet. Sometimes we have to temper our truth with kindness, and other times we have to strengthen our kindness with truth. Sometimes we have to stand up for ourselves and other times we have to soften ourselves.

Here are two aphorisms for your contemplation:

Give as much truth as kindness can bear;

and

Give as much kindness as truth can bear.

Thought creates a *container* for feeling, a shape that holds an appropriate kind of feeling. When I say, 'I am a loser', that gives a very bad feeling. These words hold bad feeling. If I say, 'I'm okay. I'm a star', that holds good feeling. Shaivism calls this the knowledge of *matrika*; the endlessly interesting study of how language shapes Consciousness and affects our inner state.

The more truth we think, feel and express, the greater energy we have. It is a first principle of Shaivism that when you lose energy, Shakti, it must be because you have strayed from truth. You may express something that seems true, but if you are moving away from energy, from the heart, from Shakti, it demonstrates that in actuality you are moving away from truth. An enlivened mantra and valid spiritual ideas have uplifting energy. Negative thoughts have a depressed energy.

UPWARD SHIFT AND DOWNWARD SHIFT

Now we come to a pair of technical terms in the inquiry we do: upward shift and *downward shift*. You hear them here in the ashram all the time. The concept of a downward shift can be used accusingly: 'I had a downward shift when you said that!' Sometimes I think I've created a monster.

These terms are self-evident: something happens or is said and we are uplifted or cast down. As we observe ourselves carefully, we go through a series of upward shifts and downward shifts. It is good to be aware of them and to observe them.

Since they are movements in Consciousness, they have something to tell us. They always have a cause. They reflect the way we interact with things. This is where inquiry takes place—where the rubber meets the road. The little *matrikas*, the almost unconscious thoughts we have, affect us.

A-STATEMENTS

Here, O monks, a monk, while experiencing a pleasant sensation, knows properly, 'I am experiencing a pleasant sensation'; while experiencing an unpleasant sensation, he knows properly, 'I am experiencing an unpleasant sensation'; while experiencing a neither-pleasant-nor-unpleasant sensation, he knows properly, 'I am experiencing a neither-pleasant-nor-unpleasant sensation'.

Gautama, the Buddha

My main topic in this lecture is what I call the A-Statement. The A-Statement is an accurate statement (A is for Accurate): an accurate statement of present feeling.

As William Carlos Williams says on being present in his poem 'Thursday':

I have had my dream—like others—
and it has come to nothing, so that
I remain now carelessly
with feet planted on the ground
and look up at the sky –
feeling my clothes about me,

the weight of my body in my shoes,
the rim of my hat, air passing in and out
at my nose—and decide to dream no more.

What does an A-Statement do? It locates where you are emotionally in this moment. A mnemonic summary of feelings is 'I feel mad, sad, bad, scared or glad'. It is Zen-like because in Zen they are mistrustful of abstract thought. If you give a Zen master a complex thought, he will hit you—*whack!* He simply wants you to be present to the moment. An A-Statement also puts you into witness-consciousness by creating a space between your awareness and the experience.

Someone recently called my attention to recent research in the field of social cognitive neuroscience at UCLA. Psychologists found that when emotions were verbally labelled (as in an A-Statement), the intensity of painful feelings diminished. The brain imaging study found that when people see a photograph of an angry or fearful face, they have increased activity in the amygdala, a part of the brain which serves as an alarm in times of danger. When the subjects verbalised the feeling shown in the photograph, like 'angry' or 'fearful', the amygdala became less active, and the right side of the brain became more active. This region, behind the forehead and eyes, has been associated with processing emotions, and thinking in words about emotional experiences.

They found that when we put feelings into words, we seem to be 'hitting the brakes' on our emotional responses. As a result, we feel less angry or fearful or sad. Similarly, by making an A-Statement, we become calmer and more grounded.

I arrived at the importance of the A-Statement as a result of a number of insights and experiences. One was a rather odd Buddhist meditation I did for a period. In it, you tried to be aware of everything you did, and verbalised it to yourself. If you were eating, you would think: 'Lifting, lifting ... placing, placing ... chewing, chewing ... swallowing, swallowing ...' As you went on eating, you would continue to say this: 'scooping, scooping ... lifting, lifting... chewing, chewing ... swallowing, swallowing ...' Your brain gave a commentary as you performed actions, a really boring kind of Andy Warhol commentary.

Instead of sitting there eating and fantasising, or worrying, I became present to the process of eating. It brought my mind into the present—where my foot is, there I am. Where my hand is, there I am.

Earlier, I described an experience I had sitting with my Guru. I had been straining for spiritual attainment and I was making myself miserable with the intensity of my yearning. Suddenly, an understanding came to me in this form: 'I can't always have the meditation I want, but I can always have the meditation I am having.'

TRACK 6. CONTEMPLATION: YOU CAN ALWAYS HAVE THE MEDITATION YOU ARE HAVING

Sit down and look within. Whatever you experience, pleasant or unpleasant, is what is given. This is the meditation you are having. Shaivism says every thought, every feeling, even every contraction is Shiva.

If you can make a verbal A-Statement, do so. If not, simply 'be as you are' in this existential moment. Say to yourself, 'I am this form of Shiva' or 'I am Shiva in this form' or 'All this is Shiva' or, as Popeye would say, 'I yam what I yam'.

Meditate with this awareness—your present experience is Shiva. As you do this, you honour your present experience. You do not reject it in favour of some imagined 'better' experience. You do not compare it with other possible meditations or with the meditation the person next to you is having. You simply have the meditation you are having, knowing that it is Shiva.

At the beginning, your acceptance of your present state might be tainted by the hope that Shiva will reward you by taking it away and revealing something more profound. Gradually you let that thought go and settle into your present experience. As you relax into it, it will reveal your deeper nature to you.

This method gives peace because it eliminates the phantom of the better meditation and the higher state we're always seeking. 'You can always have the meditation you are having' is a meditative technique you can use forever.

This understanding made me feel happy. The universe is a big and problematic place, and to get what you want from the universe moment to moment is difficult. But to surrender to what *is*, is simpler and much more sensible. To get what you want, you may have to move the whole universe. But if you surrender, you don't have to move anything but your own attitude. I said to myself, 'Have the meditation you are having'. That was good. It is a kind of A-Statement, simply being aware of what is happening, of what *is*. And letting it be as it is.

On another occasion, I had a meditation experience in which I inwardly asked what the secret of freedom and happiness is. In the inner realm, I received the extremely intriguing answer, 'When you're happy, say you're happy, and when you're sad, say you're sad. That is the way to be free'. These are really A-Statements. I was being taught to continually give myself A-Statements, to always locate myself in what is so, to be aware of what is arising.

I have said that an A-Statement is a statement of simple, present feeling. While that is true in its most pristine sense, in practice, an A-Statement is any statement that attempts to get as close as possible to present experience. Thus, 'I feel sad' is an A-Statement but so is 'I feel sad because that critic did not like my essay'. These more complex A-Statements that contain story and anecdote are valuable when dealing with actual life situations. Sometimes the simple statement of present feeling is a doorway to a more complex kind of A-Statement that brings out the details of a situation.

An A-Statement is the first plateau: base camp. Kashmir Shaivism tells us that it is okay to be where you are. Why is that? *Na shivam vidyate kvacit*: 'There is nothing that is not Shiva.' Everything is Shiva or supreme Consciousness. Every thought is Shiva, every feeling is Shiva, every mood is Shiva, *everything* is Shiva. This is the teaching of Shaivism. Clearly, it must be okay to be where you are, because wherever you are, you are in Shiva. You cannot get away from Shiva. Everything happens *within Consciousness*.

When you fight against where you are, and you are at war with the present, you are fighting Shiva. You are rejecting one part of Shiva in the belief that another part of Shiva is better. Here is the importance of the A-Statement: it is a kind of worship, a *puja*, to the sacredness of what *is*. It simply records, 'Here I am, I am sad'. There is nothing wrong with being sad. So many great poems have been written out of sadness. So many great souls have been sad. Goethe was sometimes sad. The Dalai Lama gets sad. So many great souls ... Even Lord Shiva must feel sad occasionally. He does. Immediately after creating the universe, He felt very sad. First He felt ecstatic and then He felt sad.

Let's try to make some A-Statements.

TRACK 7. INQUIRY: MAKING A-STATEMENTS

Go inside. Say to yourself, 'I feel ...'—mad, sad, bad, scared or glad. It might be a mixture of things. You might feel a cocktail of emotions. Don't worry or torment yourself about accuracy. Make an A-Statement in this moment: 'I feel ...'—let the word come to you, then fit it to the feeling and see if it seems true. Then make the A-Statement to yourself. Feel what it is like to make an A-Statement.

Here are some examples of A-Statements:

- I feel afraid.

- I feel angry.

- I'm bored.

- I want ...

- I feel restless.

- I feel depressed.

- I feel hopeless.

- I feel peaceful.

- I feel happy.

- I feel energised.

You can always bring yourself to the present by making an A-Statement.

For more A-Statements, see Appendix A.

The A-Statement, therefore, lets go of judgment of present feeling. The earth carries all kinds of beings, without judgment. It gives support equally to Mother Theresa and Hitler. In universal Consciousness, every possibility exists. Moral judgment or any kind of judgment does not enter into the picture.

Group-inquiry, as we will explore later, must be non-judgmental to allow the truth to emerge. Where our judgments are strong, possibilities are eliminated. Although each individual participant carries their own judgments, the group as a whole cancels or neutralises these judgments. It is thus closer to the character of universal Consciousness.

Something to be aware of in the area of judgment is this: the desire to eliminate judgment is itself judgmental. Judgment, too, has a place in Shiva's universe, and can and does arise in Consciousness. A perfectly good A-Statement is 'I feel judgmental'. Here, as everywhere else, a specific feeling or attitude is not a problem. It becomes a problem when it operates or motivates us unconsciously. It is right and proper to be judgmental about bad things. Thus, even if the earth does not judge Hitler, we can. You should know when you are feeling judgment and know also that there is a higher point of view as well

CLOSE YOUR EYES. WHERE'S THE FEELING?

Inquiry says, don't run away from the feeling. Turn towards the feeling, acknowledge it and inquire into it. To arrive at the A-Statement, close your eyes and ask yourself, 'Where's the feeling?' Once located, you ask, 'What feeling is this?' At the core of that feeling is bliss, is peace, is truth, is Consciousness. If you inquire into it, you peel the onion and get to the heart of the matter.

It is silly to say, 'This world is an illusion' and then still be depressed. When you say, 'I should be detached', you experience an inner war between where you want to be and where you actually are. It is good to simply locate yourself in present feeling by means of an A-Statement. It is an act of humility and closer to the truth than wishing you were somewhere else.

The A-Statement enters where the rubber meets the road. It is non-judgmental. We struggle. We say, 'I'm not where I should be'.

The A-Statement doesn't say, 'I'm angry and I shouldn't be angry'. That involves self-hatred or a tearing thought. The A-Statement says, 'I am where I am'. That is good enough. I am not going to fight and dishonour where I am. I will be one with it. I will acknowledge it. This is real self-acceptance. An A-Statement is a reality check. It is true spiritual integrity to be willing to be where you are and acknowledge it. To pretend to be 'higher' than you are is not good yoga, but, on the contrary, is simply fraud.

Once a man was travelling through the countryside and he stopped for directions from a farmer. He asked, 'How do I get to Wagga Wagga?' The farmer scratched his head and contemplated for a long time. Finally, he said, 'You can't get there from here'. It sounds reasonable but of course it is completely preposterous!

The truth is, and it is a profound truth, you can get *anywhere* from here! But if you don't know that you are *here*, you will have trouble getting somewhere else. You have to know where you are to get to the next place.

An A-Statement is useful because it points out where you really are—not where you *think* you are. It doesn't give the story of where you are, but the fact of where you *actually* are, emotionally, in this moment. You may seek transformation and inner change, but for that to happen, you have to know where you are in the first place.

With your permission, I will give you a golf analogy. You drive the ball into the woods—there is terrible emotional pain involved in that. And then you find the ball: there it is under a twig. You are still suffering over the horror that has just happened.

Now, what you have to do is be present *now*—forget the outcome of the last shot—there is a best shot playable *now*. You are in the woods. Well, Ben Hogan has been in the woods. Tiger Woods goes in the woods. They all go in the woods! They've all been there. Maybe less frequently than you do, but still, what's the essential difference?

Now you have to be present to the shot at hand, the task at hand. If you hold the ideal that you should get a three here, then you are in trouble because you will flagellate yourself with that goal. Instead, you should simply play the best possible shot. This is what it means to be present—make an A-Statement: 'I'm in the woods, I play my shot.'

The first fruit of Self-inquiry is to know where you stand. To be present: 'I am in Mt Eliza. I am in the *satsang* hall. I am with all of you. I am here.' Already, there is an intensification of awareness. When you are really angry, you may lash out at someone. But to say, 'I am angry' is to bring a little awareness in, a witness, some space. You are not so caught up.

The A-Statement points to the feeling state, which is existential rather than mental. It separates the story from the feeling. Your A-Statement might be 'I feel depressed'. Someone asks, 'Why are you depressed? You say, 'Oh, well ...' and you tell the story. In a real sense, that is not the reason for it at all. You are simply depressed because you are depressed. Depression is happening.

When you make an A-Statement, you separate from the story and you stay with the feeling itself. This is a better, more effective way to deal with it, because the story holds the ignorance that made you depressed in the first place.

An A-Statement ties thought to feeling and is more trustworthy than the thoughts that come from the feeling. When you make an A-Statement, your consciousness rises. Even though there are other statements beyond the A-Statement, as we will see, it is possible that the A-Statement is the most important one of all. This is because it locates you.

If, for example, you are angry but you are not aware of it and do not acknowledge it, then when you speak, it is actually your anger speaking. When a person is drunk and speaks wildly, people say, 'The alcohol is speaking'. When you are angry, your anger is speaking. Your anger judges everything, your anger spills out in all directions; it does damage. It would be better if you said, 'I feel angry' and you didn't push it out.

Once you become aware that you are holding anger, you can purify it and return to peace. Then your interactions are uplifting. If you are angry at a person, you say, 'You are this! You are that!' You serve them all the things you have saved up for years. Now, that is not the real truth. The real truth is simply, 'I am angry'. What you have shared with the person is the 'angry truth', which is not a high level of truth.

Similarly, with physical pain, it works better to hold it in our awareness. Pain creates fear: we won't be able to stand it; it will never go away. But when we turn our attention towards it, rather than escaping, a shift happens. The terrifying pain becomes bearable sensation in the moment. Our fear was the main problem, and must be addressed by A-Statements like 'I'm afraid I won't be able to stand this. It will never go away. This pain is so big, I will be obliterated by it'.

You might ask about the A-Statement, why do we go to feeling and not thought? We do so because feeling grounds us in the present moment. Feeling is always present. Thought travels through the whole universe. Thought goes to the future, the past, makes systems and embroiders. Of all the modalities of the psyche, only the thinking function takes us away from the present. Thinking is the very definition of being unpresent. However, in this moment, you are incontestably feeling what you are feeling. And when you are not feeling that, you are feeling something else. Feeling brings you present. And when you get in touch with the feeling, you can find the thought that is behind it, too.

The other day I was reading an essay by a well-known writer. The rational argument of it was in a certain direction but I could feel the emotion seething under the surface. I felt the author was saying something more than, or different from, his rational argument. Immediately I thought, 'What are the A-Statements?' I picked them out and wrote them down. Now I understood the text. The writer was hurt and angry and was trying to justify himself. I felt much closer to understanding the essay than I had been.

In the ashram, I have sometimes heard students comment while studying a text, 'What are the A-Statements?' In such moments, I feel proud of them because I understand that they are looking for the deeper, or the real, meaning.

POSITIVE SELF-INQUIRY

Self-inquiry is generally a negative method, stripping away the false to reveal the true. It is also possible to practise a positive method of inquiry in which the blocks or tensions are not the focus, but, instead, attention is put on the flow or the upward shift of energy.

INQUIRY: LOOKING FOR THE FOOTPRINT OF THE SELF

Turn within and look for evidence of the Self. The Self can show up in many ways, as love, as energy, as vision, as insight, as expansion, as certainty, as wonder, as peace and so on. Find the footprint of the Self and dwell on it. Relax into it. Let the sense of the Self grow and speak to you.

B- AND G-STATEMENTS

Once we get to the place of A-Statements in our inquiry, the next step is the B-Statement. B is for Beneficial. A B-Statement is 'a possibly uplifting statement'. B-Statements are the set of all possibly uplifting statements. For example, if you have a really good grandmother, she will be filled with B-Statements: 'Have some chicken soup. You're a wonderful person. You're just marvellous.' These are consoling and supportive commonsense statements. For a selection of B-Statements, see Appendix B.

A special category of B-Statements, I call G-Statements. They are scriptural statements and relate to higher Consciousness. If Grandma were Lord Shiva, she would give B-Statements like 'You are Consciousness. You are *satchitananda*' (being-Consciousness-bliss). These are G-Statements. Every religion has its own set of G-Statements, and if you want to understand the mystical core of any religion, you must find its G-Statements.

The G in G-Statement refers to God or Guru or Greatness. These are statements that originally come from a higher source. Humanity possesses a fund of these statements that have been channelled by sages and found in scripture. They uplift us. Historically, Shankaracharya was perhaps the first to appreciate the G-Statement; that is, that the essence of a whole philosophy could be summed up in one dynamic aphorism. He gathered four of these 'great statements' (*mahavakyas*) from the *Upanishads*; two of them are: *Aham Brahmasmi*: 'I am the Absolute' and *Tat tvam asi*: 'You are That.' Some Shaivite G-Statements are *Shivo'ham*: 'I am Shiva' or 'Everything is Consciousness.' For more Shaivite G-Statements, see Appendix C.

It should be noted that a G-Statement is not wishful thinking or airy-fairy. It refers to a dimension of our being that is as real and, spiritually considered, more real than our practical identity.

In defining B- and G-Statements, I use the term 'possibly uplifting' advisedly. A B-Statement for me may not be a B-Statement for you. A B-Statement that works for me today may not work for me tomorrow. A B-Statement has to have some reference to our path through life for it to be relevant, and a G-Statement has to be within reach of our current spiritual understanding.

G-STATEMENTS AND VIJNANABHAIRAVA

The seeds of the idea of the G-Statement were planted by my study of the Shaivite text *Vijnanabhairava*. This is a fascinating compendium of 112 different contemplative meditations. Each is called a *dharana*. Some of these *dharanas* take a spiritual idea, like 'All this is my own Self' or 'Everything is Consciousness' and use it as a meditative vehicle to experience the Self.

I led many workshops based on this text, and they taught me the difference between using a spiritual idea intellectually, and using it spiritually as a *dharana*. An idea like 'All this is my own Self' can be traced intellectually. A scholar might show how it developed from other ideas. A religionist might assert it as a dogma, using it as a weapon against non-believers. As a *dharana*, however, it connects one to the Self by the inward means of meditation or contemplation.

The *dharana* as presented in the *Vijnanabhairava* is precisely what I would come to describe as a G-Statement. I saw that each path and each religion had a collection of G-Statements that were the heart and soul of that path. From a certain point of view, it could be said that a religion is nothing but a fund of particular G-Statements. Such statements can be used as dogma but their real function is to elevate. They are statements of divine grace that connect us to the divinity within. The more a path or religion is filled with genuine G-Statements, the closer it is to the truth. Years of mundane intellectualising have, however, tended to obscure the mystical core of the major religions.

That each philosophy consists of a fund of G-Statements can be demonstrated by the following inquiry.

INQUIRY: PLURAL PERSPECTIVES

Go inside and locate the contraction, toxicity, tension or second force. We'll call it toxicity here. Make the A-Statement 'I feel toxic'. Then feel where your toxicity is located. Samkhya says, 'I separate from my toxicity'. Kashmir Shaivism says, 'All this toxicity is a play of Consciousness'. Vedanta says, 'All this toxicity is unreal'. Raja yoga says, 'I push this toxicity away'. *Bhakta* yoga says, 'I love toxicity'. *Hathapaka* says, 'I digest toxicity. I burn it to sameness'. Try on each of these quirky G-Statements separately and see which works.

G-STATEMENTS: MEDICINE FOR DOGMATIC THINKING

An important aspect of the G-Statement is its provisional and practical nature. As I've said, a G-Statement is really a G-Statement only when it *functions* as a G-Statement; that is, it uplifts the practitioner. You might take the most hallowed of G-Statements like 'Everything is Shiva' or 'Jesus loves you' but if it doesn't help the meditator in that moment, then, for that person, it is not functionally a G-Statement.

Recently, one of my students told me about a Shiva Process Self-inquiry private session he did with a young woman. She had a contraction in her navel chakra. At a certain point in the process, he gave her the G-Statement (in the form of a prayer), 'God, please help me when I get overwhelmed'. This increased the contraction. My student intelligently saw that this called for a different approach. He suggested, 'God, please give me more strength and self-control'. That released the contraction.

It is important to observe that there was nothing wrong with the original G-Statement, except that it situationally didn't work. And, similarly, there was nothing inherently superior about the second one, except that it did work. It is interesting to contemplate the implications of the difference between the two statements. We could arrive at the hypothesis that her inner being found the second statement empowering because it put her self-development in her own hands. I'll emphasise again, though, that the first statement, marked by a devotional attitude of surrender, might work for another person.

Understanding the provisional nature of the G-Statement gave me an insight into the path of Vedanta, with which I had long wrestled. I had always felt troubled by the Vedantic idea, 'This whole world is an illusion', when it was asserted as fundamental truth or dogma. But I subsequently had no trouble accepting that the teaching 'This whole world is an illusion' could *sometimes* function as an uplifting G-Statement. In fact, I occasionally found it useful.

In the same way, the hoary conflict between Buddhism and Hinduism, the non-Self versus the Self, can be sidestepped when we take on the concept of the G-Statement. The idea of emptiness is a useful meditative tool, even for one who holds the idea of the 'Self'. Seen this way, both the theory of emptiness and the theory of the Self are useful methods, and not mutually exclusive. Later, I will talk about the process of feedback in group-inquiry. It is very much in the spirit of Shiva Process that apparently antithetical G-Statements like 'I am the Self' and 'There is no Self' can be offered one after the other. Both are 'possibly uplifting'. All the G-Statements gathered by the different paths and religions must have worked for some people in some context. Therefore, all should be respected and regarded as part of a pharmacopoeia of G-Statements; medicine for different diseases. Genuine Self-inquiry cannot be aligned with a specific dogma or religious belief, as we saw in the previous inquiry. It must be part of the philosophy of Consciousness, which includes everything.

The proper function of a G-Statement is its use as a meditative instrument of *sadhana* or connection to a higher truth. It is a perversion of a G-Statement to use it dogmatically. Since no spiritual concept can be the same as the Absolute, the Absolute is always beyond any idea, no matter how glorious. Otherwise, universal Consciousness could be held within the bounds of a thought-form, and that is clearly self-contradictory.

Our awareness is usually so scattered and so not 'on purpose' that when we inject a G-Statement into it, it focuses attention in a beneficial way. Consciousness is thrown towards its centre, if only for a moment. And the effect of that is to quiet the mind and uplift the spirit.

INQUIRY: TURNING A-STATEMENTS INTO G-STATEMENTS

I have said that each A-Statement honours a mood of Shiva. You can lift A-Statements from being trapped in the personal by turning them into G-Statements.

First, get in touch with present feeling. Make your A-Statement. Instead of saying, 'I feel angry' or 'I feel happy', or whatever you feel, say, 'Shiva is angry' or 'Shiva is happy'. What we just did is turn an A-Statement into a G-Statement.

TRACK 8. CONTEMPLATION: G-STATEMENTS

Read the following G-Statements. They are either directly from the Shaivite scriptures or glossed from them. With each one, you should watch how they impact you. See if they are easy to accept or not, and notice where they affect you. Do they go into your heart, your third eye? Do they uplift you? See if any of them open up a doorway within you. In these G-Statements, 'Shiva' is synonymous with the Self, God, or universal Consciousness.

- Everything is Consciousness.

- Consciousness is the most healing and desirable thing.

- I am Shiva.

- Every thought and feeling, even my blocks, are Shiva.

- The way I think creates the experience of my life.

- This universe is drenched in love.

- I am the Lord of Matrika.

- There is absolutely no problem.

- All these people are Shiva in their own universe.

- Everything is perfect as it is.

- Whatever meditation I am having is Shiva.

PRACTISING SELF-INQUIRY

The process of Self-inquiry, then, consists of first locating yourself—through A-Statements, then exploring and uplifting through B- and G-Statements. You may want to get into a mind-free state, but, in fact, the voice in your mind is always making statements. There is a script going on, there is a narrator in there. It's talking, it's saying, it's speaking, it's shrinking, it's expanding, it's commenting. Constant mental activity takes place, including tearing thoughts, wishful thoughts and inflated thoughts.

The mind is untrained and unkempt and it needs to be disciplined. It has to move in the right direction, to the awareness of A-Statements and then on to B- and G-Statements.

Sometimes I wonder why we were designed this way. Why did the Lord put a voice inside of us that afflicts us like this? I wasn't there at the time or I would have talked Him out of it. I would have said, 'Please don't put that voice in there! And if you do have to put a voice in, use good CDs, not tearing thoughts'.

When Adam and Eve ate the apple, they experienced the first tearing thoughts. Before they ate it, their life in the Garden of Eden was perfect. There were no tearing thoughts. Scholars call that period of perfection in Eden 'prelapsarian'; before the 'lapse'. Then guilt arose, along with tearing thoughts.

That was the fall of humanity. The unhappy couple had to leave Eden, where they had lived in timeless bliss. We are their children, living in the horror created by the workings of our own minds. Through inquiry, we can pull the rug out from those tearing thoughts and find Eden again.

Catholic theology has an interesting concept called *felix culpa*, the 'fortunate fall'. From this perspective, that means there was a silver lining to the fall in the garden because it allowed Jesus to come later and redeem us.

Perhaps we can say, by analogy, it is good that we fell from innocence so we can do *sadhana* with enthusiasm, and recapture our Shiva nature. An infant is pure and innocent and in touch with the Divine, but to become enlightened, it must suffer a fall into separation and then reclaim its connectedness as an adult.

THE STEPS OF PERSONAL INQUIRY

For handy reference, I will now give a practical overview of personal inquiry, which you can adapt to your practice. I will also outline the steps of inquiry in specific areas of life.

PERSONAL INQUIRY

1. Turn within and discover tension or second force in the navel, heart, throat and third eye.

2. Ask what emotion this is. Is it anger, fear or sadness?

3. Make A-Statements.

4. Ask inside what caused this.

5. Inquire what can be done to overcome this.

6. Make B-Statements.

7. Make G-Statements resolving the situation spiritually. I recommend that if at any point in the process you obtain a significant upward shift and diminution of tension, be satisfied with that and end the inquiry and meditate.

INQUIRY INTO SPECIFIC AREAS OF LIFE

The following method is similar except it focuses on a specific area of life: body, career, relationship or spirituality. Self-inquiry is an extremely plastic technique that can be used universally to unblock inner obstacles. Thus, you can do inquiry into a specific work situation or relationship issue, even an upcoming event that you're helping to plan.

1. Turn within.

2. Select the area of life which most needs investigation (body, career, relationship or spirituality).

3. Bring that area of life into your inner world in a general way without being too concrete, and notice any reaction that happens in the four chakras: the navel, heart, throat and third eye.

4.　　If a tension or second force shows up, process it as in Personal Inquiry (see Steps 1–7) in relation to the area of life under inquiry.

For a series of Self-inquiry questions on areas of life, play Track 15 or see Appendix D.

TRACK 9. INQUIRY: PERSONAL INQUIRY

- Look within. Scan the four chakras* for tension.

- Find where you hold the most tension or second force.

- Give yourself A-Statements until you are satisfied that you have accurately described the feeling.

- Give yourself B- and G-Statements until a shift occurs.

- Meditate.

*For a full outline of the Self-Inquiry Guided Chakra Meditation, play Track 1 or see Appendix E.

TRACK 10.
INQUIRY: ADVANCED PERSONAL INQUIRY

This is a streamlined version of personal inquiry for adept meditators:

- Discover where you hold the most second force, and make A-Statements.

- Keeping in mind that any second force or tension you hold is based on some sort of wrong understanding, ask yourself, 'What do I have to do to shift this feeling?'

THE STUDY OF CONSCIOUSNESS

Shiva Process is the study of Consciousness. By Consciousness, I don't mean only mental consciousness, I mean the heart and the mind together. It is the study of the laws of your inner world. The A-, B- and G-Statements are techniques we have evolved. They are very good techniques, but there could be other techniques. There could be a whole different Shiva Process that would work as well. In fact, I believe that Self-inquiry is at the cutting edge of the evolution of Consciousness, and that would imply that there are other versions of the Shiva Process in play even as I speak. But for this method and for any of the other methods that might or might not be out there, the goal to understand Consciousness is the same.

Consciousness has laws and you discover them as you inquire. Every spiritual person must study their own awareness. You must study the laws of your heart and your mind—how they open and close, expand and contract. You have to study that. Of course, when I say 'study', I'm using it in the sense of spiritual or internal education, which I call *Second Education*, whereas *First Education* is conventional education of the intellect and personality. Second Education is not an intellectual pursuit, but the search for wisdom and happiness. First Education focuses mainly on information, overlooking the important elements of feeling and energy. The technical elements I've discussed are simply the particular lenses that we use here, but the essence is the study of awareness: being aware of awareness, moment to moment.

If tomorrow, some better techniques come along, we'll take them. Shiva Process is a minestrone. We take whatever is useful, whatever is a good investigative tool, and throw it into the soup.

QUESTIONS AND ANSWERS

THE FOUR CENTRES

Question: Why do we use only four of the classical seven chakras?
Swamiji: The four centres we investigate are more like Gurdjieff's centres: the moving centre (navel), the emotional centre (heart),

and the intellectual centre (third eye), plus communication central (throat). They also relate to Vital (navel), Peculiar (heart) and Solid (third eye).

We could use the seven chakras as a way of gathering information, but our method seems to yield the best results. As far as the *sahasrara* (crown of the head) goes, it's well worth meditating on that place. As I mentioned earlier, it is transpersonal, while the personal issues are all lower down. The four centres we use tend to be where people experience their blocks. Of course, if someone notices a fierce contraction lower than the navel, that can be investigated.

DEALING WITH TEARING THOUGHTS

Question: My problem is that I believe my tearing thoughts. I don't know how to get around this. It's hard to oppose them when I actually believe them.

Swamiji: Everyone is susceptible to their own choice group of tearing thoughts. If you didn't believe them, they wouldn't be tearing thoughts. What you have to do is develop a new criterion for validation. Normally, you have a tearing thought like 'I'm a loser', and then you validate it by pointing to horrible calamities in your life. When you try to oppose it, the bad outweighs the good, and the tearing thoughts win. You need a different criterion, which is your inner feeling. When you allow your tearing thoughts to win, you feel miserable. And since you know that you are the Self, that can't be right. You reject your tearing thoughts because they make you feel contracted and miserable, and for no 'objective criterion'. Please understand what I'm saying. You are free to reject ways of telling yourself your own story that deplete and contract you. You are free to tell yourself your own story in a way that gives you Shakti.

Question: I sense that there is some tearing thought under all my tearing thoughts that I can't quite get to. Does this make sense to you?

Swamiji: That's a good insight. You could call it a basic tearing thought. In Shaivism, they call it *anava mala*; the basic limiting condition. It's a kind of foundational thought that is your custom-made Achilles heel. If you can ferret it out and stare it down, you've done well. Then you have to focus on the opposite.

What you describe will feel so much a part of you that you can hardly imagine life without it. Usually, this kind of tearing thought is outside your conscious awareness and it hangs around your inner world like a toxic soup. It can be the sense, 'I am a loser' or 'I'll never get what I want' or 'I'm unlovable'. You get the idea. When you get to this level of *anava mala*, you will discover how much of your psychic world is dominated by this basic thought. The truth is that you can live very well without it and, also, you can overcome it. Once you do, it's almost as though you have had an incarnation change. You are simply not the same person any more. And thank God for that (but don't be offended)!

Question: To what extent should you articulate tearing thoughts in inquiry?

Swamiji: There are two points of view implicit here. You could ask, why involve yourself in any suffering if you can avoid it? And who could argue with that? But the other point of view is also compelling. It says that the descent into hell is good as long as it doesn't ruin you. It's the 'school of experience' point of view: anything that doesn't kill you makes you stronger. From this perspective, finding your actual tearing thoughts and witnessing their effect inside you is excellent. You get to see how negative they are and to observe where your weaknesses lie. Again, the assumption is that in doing so, you don't lose your connection with the Self and become undone.

Let's say your worst tearing thought is 'I'm unlovable, no one cares about me'. It's good to meet it face to face and to see its effect on you. However, you will observe that when you simply say, 'I'm having tearing thoughts', there's a much better feeling and you short-circuit that particular mire.

Maybe I belong to the school of experience—I think it's good to know the face of your enemy, but you don't have to go there again and again.

TELL THE TRUTH AND DON'T GET ANGRY

Question: I can relate to your discussion of truth and kindness. I think that I go into both red zones; that is, I sometimes get angry and say too much, and at other times I don't speak up.

Swamiji: This is a razor's edge for everyone. The dharma of telling the truth and not getting angry is really useful. I suggest you approach these issues in meditation. Inquire within: 'In what areas or situations in life do I suppress my communication? Where in my life is my communication blocked?' Always investigate the most obvious things first, the biggest blocks. Once you locate an area of life, then get in touch with the feeling that you carry about it. Let's say it's a feeling of tension in the navel or the throat—then, using the methods of Self-inquiry, go right into the feeling and work until you come to peace.

This can also be approached retrospectively; that is, make a review of your day and inquire whether any of your communications or encounters featured suppressed communication or overabundant angry communication. Investigate the feeling that comes up and rewrite the script in your imagination, bringing yourself to peace.

BEING PRESENT WITH A-STATEMENTS

Question: Sometimes I become aware that I feel bad and I don't know why or how it happened—any advice?

Swamiji: The bad feeling is like a footprint in the sand. It has a cause and that cause is discoverable. Something must have happened, you must have had a reaction to something. Always begin with the A-Statement, get as close to the present feeling as you can and try to be content with simply being with the present feeling.

When you relax into it and sit with it, it will start to tell you what you need to know. Or if it doesn't tell you anything, then just be with it. In itself, that can cause a shift, even if you don't discover the source of the bad feeling.

Question: How can I use A-Statements in my inquiry?

Swamiji: It is good to make A-Statements within yourself, in your own inner world. In fact, you might give yourself the assignment, 'Just make A-Statements all the time'. Then you will constantly record where you are, without trying to change anything. It is a form of self-observation. You can do it silently. It brings you to the present moment.

In the old factories, workers used to use conveyor belts. They would do the same operation to each object that came in front of them. Then the belt would move along and bring up the next one. Your feelings are on a conveyor belt. If you do the operation of making an A-Statement to the feeling of the moment, then the next moment might bring a new feeling. It might not, but in some moment, inevitably, it will.

Question: I am filled with the most vile emotions. I try to say my mantra intensely to move away from them, or think about pure Consciousness. I think that if I did inquiry, I would be inundated by lust, greed and jealousy; that is my doubt.

Swamiji: My Guru had a big struggle with lust. He thought he had conquered it and then it arose forcibly at an advanced stage in his meditation. These emotions are part of our psyche, and they actually gain power when we try to control them by force or suppression. A great sage taught my Guru how to overcome lust by transforming it into acceptance. You could take refuge in the A-Statement.

No one has lust every second. When it rises up, make the A-Statement, 'I have lust'. Similarly, when appropriate, say:

I feel greedy.

I am angry.

I am full of desire.

I am afraid.

I feel jealous.

I feel grief.

When you acknowledge each of these things, they will come and go, and you won't create resistance, which perpetuates them. When you become one with whatever is arising, you create the conditions in which change can take place; you restore the flow.

Question: Sometimes when I try to find my A-Statements, I get to a certain level that seems true and then I realise there's a deeper reality. For example, I recently thought 'I am bored' and then on continued investigation I discovered 'I am angry' and 'I am sad' underneath the boredom. When do you stop deconstructing your A-Statements?

Swamiji: In a sense, you never do because Consciousness is an infinite ocean. And it's also true that some complex emotions like boredom are constructed of simpler ones. If you think outside the box for a moment, you'll see that underneath your 'I am angry' and 'I am sad', there's a deeper 'A-Statement'—'I am Shiva'. The A-Statement of God is 'I am God' or 'I am Consciousness' or 'Om'. The ultimate A-Statement is the sound the universe makes in its own Self-knowing. From below, this would be a G-Statement, but from Shiva's perspective, it's His A-Statement. Never stop investigating until you find the pot of gold. But as a practical guideline, when you feel a palpable shift, you should know that you've completed at least that part of the work.

EMOTION AND FEELING

Question: Is there a difference between emotion and feeling?

Swamiji: The state of the Self is feeling, thinking, doing—*iccha, jnana, kriya* in Shaivite terms. Sometimes we think of nirvana as being a plane of Consciousness with no feeling; maybe like something from a science-fiction movie, like an abstract space or a void. A Shaivite thinks of it differently. The essence, the heart of God, of Consciousness, is energy. Divine energy has two aspects: a feeling aspect and a thinking aspect. The feeling in God is divine love, divine peace. Emotions are waves or contractions of that original feeling. Negative emotions are something like distortions of that original feeling. They are waves on the ocean of feeling—produced by wrong thinking.

Even if a negative emotion is a distortion of divine feeling, it should not be forgotten that it is essentially very close to the Divine. Thus, every negative emotion has a positive aspect. For example, anger, as destructive as it is, is also strong. That is why anger is sometimes mistaken for strength, and strength is sometimes mistaken for anger. The feeling of sadness is related to sympathy and compassion, while the feeling of fear is related to humility and perhaps openness. Knowing this, you become able to turn your negative emotions towards their positive dimension.

Question: I have a lot of problems with anger. Any suggestions?

Swamiji: Anger may be your 'chief fault'. Most of us have a particular negative emotion that is especially destructive for us. For some, it is anger; for others, it is fear or sorrow. That specific emotion robs us of our self-esteem and energy, and makes us particularly contracted.

It's good to know your chief fault and to work hard against it. Other negative emotions might be kryptonite to other people, but to you they can be a means of help. So, when you feel anger coming on, inquire if the feeling could be interpreted as fear or sadness. In this case, fear and sadness won't be bad for you, but actually good. They will take you one layer deeper and openly undermine your anger.

It's important to work hard against your chief fault. Don't worry about the other negative emotions. You can even playfully exaggerate them. When you feel anger coming up, say, 'I feel so sad' or 'I feel terrified'. Notice the effect such statements have. You might say that you're giving false A-Statements, but I have a more charitable way of looking at it. You're actually using false A-Statements as B-Statements. If you avoid indulging your chief fault, you can relish a modest excursion into other negative emotions.

WHEN A SOLUTION IS NOT AT HAND

Question: Sometimes I have a big issue I am struggling with and I feel particularly emotional about it. On some occasions, I can get to the bottom of it through Self-inquiry, but other times, no matter how hard I work, I can't solve it. Is it because I haven't found the right statement? Or should I just grit my teeth and tough it out? I am wondering what the next step is when that happens.

Swamiji: When you do inquiry, have compassion for yourself. You are not going to solve every issue instantly. There are big issues that may be many lifetimes forming—we can't master them in a moment.

Of course, major breakthroughs occur, but it also can be like the oyster with a grain of sand: it has to be worked for a long time, though it irritates you. That irritation eventually becomes a pearl. Issues that are really big can take years to gestate. Don't be impatient. There is some wisdom or some illumination that will come and change it, although it may be out of your reach in this moment. Let that be okay for you.

In such a situation, you can say, 'My ignorance is greater than my yoga at this moment'. That is fine, that is honourable, too. Lord Vishnu incarnated as a boar, a pig. He became the boar-avatar. He got down here and He was rooting around in the mud, squeaking and oinking. And He got so enamoured of the sensual joy of being in the mud that He forgot what His purpose was. He was completely caught in the mud.

Finally, His absence was noticed in the heavenly realms so Lord Shiva went down to investigate. Shiva was disgusted, seeing Lord Vishnu wallowing in forgetfulness. He stuck Him with His trident. As Lord Vishnu died, as His soul left the pig's body, He laughed as He remembered who He was! What I am saying is that it is honourable to acknowledge your present limitations even while holding your divinity in your mind. Even Lord Vishnu got trapped in maya.

Question: There is something I have wanted for a long time and it has always been blocked, no matter how hard I strive for it. I'm sure this is a common situation. Do you have any suggestions for me?

Swamiji: The first force you have is creating a lot of second force. Perhaps you can think about it this way: you shouldn't try to suppress or deny your first force. The force of desire is nothing but *kundalini*. It is a divine expression of your freedom. The problem is that sometimes we put our desire in the wrong direction. Search for a way you can use the same impulse in a new direction. I like to say, 'Don't keep pounding at locked doors; look for the open door'.

I'll give you an example from my own life. My Guru's teaching was to welcome everyone with love. He was against sectarian enmity and was for oneness. Nonetheless, after he died, his disciples split into warring factions. There was so much enmity. This one hated that one; that one hated this one. There was a great deal of mud-slinging and public calumny.

I hated this situation and did everything in my power to create oneness. I wanted there to be reconciliation and an acknowledgment of our common heritage, as well as the spirit of my Guru's teaching. I had some success through The 3 Gurus programs: local and international events hosted by three Gurus who share the spiritual tradition of Bhagawan Nityananda.

In general, however, the different factions have been locked into their hatred and self-righteousness. At some point, I allowed the situation to teach me that I had a tremendous urge for oneness and communication, and for bridging chasms of hatred and mistrust. A chain of events led me into the realm of interfaith dialogue where I found that my fire for oneness was welcomed. There, all the doors opened up and I found people who agreed with my point of view and wanted to hear my message.

CAN B-STATEMENTS INFLATE THE EGO?

Question: While doing inquiry, I have used B-Statements and have had a definite upward shift, which is great. But then afterwards, I was worried that the B-Statements actually appealed to my ego and strengthened it. I wanted to know what your perspective is from a yogic point of view.

Swamiji: Don't worry about it. Don't be hard on yourself. If you have an inflation that seems like ego in that moment, let it happen. There is a natural rhythm in things. If you think of it as a gift of the spirit, you won't get inflated. Shaivites don't worry too much about inflation because they make everything part of their relationship with the Divine. Conventional yogis are always scrutinising themselves in fear of ego, but that puts them at war with themselves.

The universe is a perfect feedback system. If the ego is inflated, it will naturally get chopped down. Don't do it yourself. Just be aware. It is good to have self-esteem. It is good to love yourself. My Guru used to say, 'Honour yourself, worship yourself, God dwells within you as you'. Ego becomes a problem when it asserts and affirms and pushes its way through. It creates second force. To feel good about yourself allows the joy to rise up; it is not ego. This is a complex issue. We have to learn to distinguish between the expansion of ego and the expansion of the Self. As always, a lot depends on attitude.

SPIRITUAL RELATIVITY

Question: I'm a Buddhist and to me your teaching on G-Statements seems very relativistic. In the Buddha's eightfold path, number one is right view, by which he meant that it is necessary to have a true spiritual philosophy to attain the goal. What if a wrong doctrine gives you an upward shift?

Swamiji: Yes, the method of feedback and the concept of G-Statements bring the traditional teachings into a new focus. Look at it this way. As I've mentioned, thousands and thousands of great Buddhist yogis have denied the existence of a permanent Self. Thousands and thousands of great Hindu yogis have affirmed the existence of a permanent Self. What should we do with this indisputable fact? Either one side is right, and the other side is completely deluded and hopelessly lost, or somehow both sides are right.

I've met great masters in both traditions, and to my eye, their attainment seemed the same, therefore I think it's true that doctrines can clash horizontally and yet meet at infinity like the proverbial parallel lines. That's why I say that you should use the G-Statements within your tradition to go deeper into the truth rather than use them as weapons against conflicting G-Statements from other traditions. We can all discuss this further in heaven. Remember, conflicts at a low level of Consciousness become resolved at a higher level.

Question: Your use of A-, B- and G-Statements hints that you have a radical view of the role of ideas. I can't quite put my finger on it; could you say something about this?

Swamiji: You must have observed that I have an extreme allergy to dogma (as I say that, I'm wondering if, by the law of opposites, it really means I'm rather dogmatic). Some modern yogis tend to take a few admittedly noble ideas and work them to death as though the truth dwelt in those ideas. It seems to me that they are guilty of reification; that is, they think of these ideas as having some kind of concrete reality. The implication of the A-, B- and G-Statement model is the relativity of all spiritual ideas. Ideas are to be used, and they are useful if they give us a positive result.

Realisation is not conceptual. It is a matter of establishing an abiding contact with the Self. Noble spiritual ideas can facilitate this goal because you can 'ride' them to the Self when conditions are right. The ideas are not inherently truthful, but they can interact with the practitioner to create a truthful result. In my view, ideas are not the goal, but are a method to achieve the goal.

The Self is always prior to ideas. A fundamentalist may say this scripture or that scripture or another scripture is the absolute word of God (and a number of scriptures have their fundamentalists), but it is the actual fundamentalist, the subject, who decides to believe that any particular scripture is the word of God. The scripture itself just lies there.

UPWARD SHIFT

Question: I am interested in the concept of the upward shift. Do you have any advice about how to study it more fully?

Swamiji: The ideal way is to observe the upward shift as it appears in nature; nature being your reaction to things. Notice what gives you an upward shift and work out why. As we practised reviewing our day in Lecture 1, looking for contractions, you can review your day before you go to sleep and ask yourself, 'Were there any upward shifts?' As you remember them, you won't always know the causes until you inquire more deeply.

If you are impatient and want to create upward shifts artificially, practise a creative meditation. For example, remember the best and most energised time of your life. Close in on the feeling of it. Observe the *matrikas*, the thought-forms, that underlay the good feeling of that time.

Be careful to focus on the inner movements and not on externals or the story. For example, if the underlying thought is 'I love Bob', that could lead to grief and nostalgia and other biographical complexities. Instead, focus on the impersonal aspect of loving Bob, like 'I am full of love'.

The important thing is to closely observe the relationship between thought and feeling, and what kinds of thoughts create the upward shift of feeling. The best ones are G-Statements that speak about our fundamental nature as Consciousness. But because we are so embroiled in our personal dramas, it sometimes works better to use elements of that drama to create the upward shift.

THE ZEN OF SELF-INQUIRY

Question: I've heard you say that Self-inquiry is similar to Zen Buddhism. Could you say something more about that?

Swamiji: It does have points of resemblance to Zen. Zen is suspicious of spiritual conceptualising and moralising. It mistrusts philosophy; it mistrusts morality. When I first did inquiry in my Guru's presence, I noticed that many spiritual ideas and explanations arose in me.

How could I know which one was true? Sometimes a thing and its opposite would both come into my mind simultaneously. Then I would think, how can I choose between these alternatives with any certainty? I guess, like Descartes, I was looking for solid ground. Thoughts and moral judgments could not provide that solid ground, but I saw that getting in touch with present experience could. Zen also asks, first of all, 'What is so?' which is an uptown version of my favourite question, 'What's going on here?'

CHILDREN'S SELF-INQUIRY

Question: Do you have any tips for teaching Self-inquiry to young children?

Swamiji: Children can do surprisingly effective Self-inquiry. However, don't expect young ones to do it on their own; you'll have to guide them. You should concentrate on the A-Statement level. To do this, ask them questions so that their awareness of their feelings increases. Once they get in touch with what they're actually experiencing, nature or the Self will take over and I think you'll find it quite delightful.

Ask them questions so their inquiry becomes more and more concrete. You can ask them where they have the feeling, whether it is big or small, and if it has a colour or a shape. Ask them what the feeling could be made of, any question that helps them get close to the feeling. Then ask them if they feel angry or sad or scared. You can even have them make an A-Statement like 'I feel angry' or 'I feel sad' or 'I feel scared'. You can ask them what the feeling is about and what thoughts, people or images come to mind.

Once you feel close to it, you can ask them how they can make the feeling better. You'll see that the process of inquiry is natural, and children will spontaneously come up with wonderful solutions. Working with your children like this will benefit them immensely because they will establish a habit of being aware of their inner responses. So, use questions, guide them along the path to awareness and, really, be content with the A-Statement level of awareness. If a shift happens, that's a bonus.

One of my students is a primary school teacher and she does the Shiva Process with her pupils, calling it 'The Sentence Game'. They simply love it. She demonstrated it to the whole school, and other staff members were impressed and could see the benefits. Instead of 'making a statement', the children were invited to 'make up a sentence'.

THE THREE TYPES

Question: What happens if you are Peculiar because you are extremely passionate and emotional? But you are also Solid, because you intellectualise everything. And then you want to go off and do things all the time, so you are Vital as well. Can you be all three? Does one waft in and out of each one?

Swamiji: It is good to be balanced in all three, because everyone is made up of all three. But, there is usually one area that we haven't developed and need to work on. We need balance on every level. I will say this about your question ... [Asks the audience:] What was his question? Solid, Vital or Peculiar? It was Peculiar, because why? It was charming, charismatic, humorous and dramatic. It had lovely Peculiar qualities. So, what do you think he is? ... The girls here—they are all certified clairvoyants, witches and seers—say that you are a Peculiar-Solid.

Situations emphasise one aspect more than others. A group of athletes will tend to be Vital, but within that group, some are more Peculiar than others. Life gives each aspect an appropriate work-out.

Question: I think I am a Peculiar and that may contribute to the fact that it's hard for me to accomplish things in life. What can a poor Peculiar do?

Swamiji: Every type has a strength but also a weakness. As you grow spiritually, the first job is to strengthen the weak part. As you suggest, Peculiars often lack Vital. It's good for Peculiars to do physical work or at least work that involves the material world. It grounds them and makes them more practical. That's why in ashrams you often see people working against their type, at least for a little while. For example, an intellectual comes to an ashram and it's clear that their ultimate service to the Guru will involve publications or library work or something of that kind. However, for a number of years they're out in the garden digging trenches (oops, I might be talking about myself here). The period of working against type creates balance.

As you say, Peculiars often lack the Vital quality. Solids often lack the Peculiar quality. That produces the 'dry intellectual': the Vulcan, Mr Spock, who is not in touch with his feeling. The Vital type most often lacks Solid. They're great at doing, but not so good at thinking. Hence, the 'dumb Vital' who charges off in a new wrong direction every day. When they balance themselves and bring in the element of discrimination, then they'll be able to make good use of their already considerable powers of doing.

It makes intuitive sense to deal with an imbalance or an excess by meditating and expanding what's lacking. So, in your case, you should meditate on the Vital. Put your awareness in your navel and think thoughts like 'I can do. I am a competent person'. See if you can get in touch with the energy of doing. And listen—you should do some physical things, too, like gardening or hiking or playing sports.

DEALING WITH PEOPLE

Question: My experiences with other people tend to be so unpleasant that I have a strong desire to go off somewhere and be a hermit. Is it possible to be too sensitive to live in society?

Swamiji: If you really look at yourself, I think you'll discover that you are not afraid of other people, but actually of your own feeling. When you admit that to yourself, you will become less afraid. It's only your own feeling after all, it won't kill you and it can be transmuted. Do the *tapasya*, the spiritual burning, of hanging in there with your own experience. Instead of running from a feeling, be with it and inquire into it. As soon as you use inquiry, you will diffuse it. Every feeling has something to teach us and offers a new insight. Under every feeling, there is a core of peace that can be attained by courageous practice.

Question: I'm clear that I want to leave a long-term relationship. As a stalwart practitioner of Self-inquiry, do I have a responsibility to communicate about it or should I just move on?

Swamiji: That's a good question. Modern culture is one of non-inquiry. War, tantrums and blame are standard ways of operating. A culture of inquiry is different. In such a culture, there is a responsibility to get to the bottom of things. Still, the law of relationships operates: either partner can unilaterally terminate it at any time. I suggest you make every attempt for a full and loving communication combining truth and kindness. You may have to say your piece and stand your ground while the other person's emotions arise—that's all right, it won't kill you. But I'd recommend that you don't submit yourself to the same thing over and over again. In the course of living, people are bound to sometimes blame you and yell at you. Sometimes it's justified and it's good to have the courage to bear it and let it pass through you. But you shouldn't have to swallow the same serve over and over again or be anointed by the same negative emotions more than once.

Question: I've found that the Shiva Process works very well for relationships, perhaps even more so than for self-knowledge. Would you agree with that?

Swamiji: From a certain perspective, spirituality is only about relationship. The perfect relationship, one in which there is no problem of duality, is the relationship of identity. When you are one with something, you don't have a problem with that thing. Thus the Vedic G-Statement 'I am Brahman' is an equal sign. It says that 'I' and 'Brahman' are one and not two things.

Our language expresses relationship. The G-Statement essentially affirms the oneness of the individual and the Divine. And language also contains energy. When language is more perfect, as in the G-Statement, it holds more energy. But when ego or separation is affirmed, then language loses energy. The more oneness you feel with others—the more human sympathy—the more exalted you become. Relationship is nothing but the path of devotion. Everyone wants to merge with the beloved. And why not? It is the highest ecstasy.

SUMMARY

- We live in two worlds—the outer world and the inner world.

- The inner world has two aspects: thought and feeling.

- Tearing thoughts lead to negative emotion.

- There are thinking, feeling and doing types.

- Look for the balance between truth and kindness.

- Look for the upward shift of energy and be alert to the downward shift.

- A-Statements locate where you are now.

- An A-Statement is a *puja* to the sacredness of what *is*.

- Feeling is always present.

- Positive Self-inquiry focuses on upward shifts instead of blocks.

- B-Statements are possibly uplifting statements.

- G-Statements are scriptural B-Statements that come from a higher source.

- A G-Statement can function as a means to connect you to God.

- G-Statements are provisional rather than dogmatic.

- Shiva Process is the study of awareness.

- Every negative emotion has a positive aspect.

- Our chief fault is a particular negative emotion that is especially destructive for us.

- Children's Self-inquiry should focus on the A-Statement.

- Ego diminishes energy.

PART II
GROUP-INQUIRY

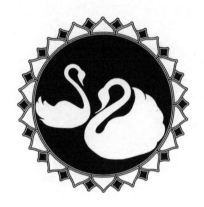

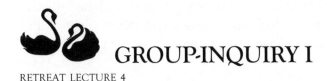 # GROUP-INQUIRY I

Inquire into the nature of truth. Abandon falsehood.
Yoga Vashishta

A friend's eye is a good looking-glass.
Gaelic Proverb

SO FAR, I have been talking about the elements of personal Self-inquiry. Now I begin a discussion of group-inquiry. When we use the elements of inquiry in a group, the fire of awareness is kindled. In the West, we can find precursors to group-inquiry in therapy groups and '60s-style encounter groups. In the East, I see an analogy with the Vedic *yagna*; a fire ritual in which priests sit around a sacred fire intoning mantras (see Lecture 5). In *Consciousness Is Everything*, I drew a parallel with the Tantric *kula-chakra* ritual. Despite these precedents, group-inquiry is a completely new twist on an old method.

You will often see writers refer to 'mind' and 'awareness' as though there were a collective understanding of what these things mean. In fact, there are many levels of awareness, many 'voices' within a person, and it is important to distinguish them. Mundane consciousness, the awareness of an ordinary person lost in the worldly struggle without recourse to spirituality, is marked by confusion and lack of a clear centre.

In that state of mind, many thoughts are generated by unconscious feelings of fear and desire. The consciousness is unexamined, unexplored and unprocessed. It is a chaos of thoughts and feelings, largely negative. It is essentially a state of suffering. Of course, pleasant states come and go but there is little rhyme or reason to them. The awareness is not under the control of the person. Ninety-nine per cent of the world lives in that state of mind, and the suffering implicit in that state is what often turns us to drugs, alcohol and the psychiatric pharmacopoeia. Fortunate ones turn towards the spiritual path.

A higher level of Consciousness is what Gurdjieff calls 'Self-remembering': an act of awareness focusing on and examining itself. By this practice—and it is a 'practice'—Consciousness is brought to a higher state, even if elements of contraction and pain are present.

In our terms, such a shift is brought about by the A-Statement. While the ordinary mind is unconscious, the A-Statement helps to makes us conscious. With it, you manifest awareness of what is happening right here and now. The A-Statement, then, is a form of Self-remembering.

A person who remembers the Self, who makes A-Statements, is a seeker. It is only seekers who start to become aware of themselves. They become aware of their previously unconscious tearing thoughts and other hidden factors. When they make good A-Statements, they become (at least briefly) calm and detached and aware. For example, you may be afflicted by the tearing thought, 'I am worthless'. Instead, you make the A-Statement, 'I am having tearing thoughts'. Notice that the statement 'I am having tearing thoughts' is true: you *are* having tearing thoughts, whereas the statement 'I am worthless' is debatable and mood-generated. The A-Statement has more energy than the tearing thought, which actually robs you of energy. That is because the A-Statement is closer to the truth.

A third level of awareness is introjection or substitution. Here, one consciously substitutes positive thoughts for negative thoughts. We might use affirmations or mantra. We enter our mental process proactively and instead of allowing it to unfold in a helter-skelter way, we work with it, transforming what we don't like. This is the level of the B-Statement. It is the level of the wise person. We are not talking about scriptural wisdom only, but also commonsense or practical wisdom. A wise person reassures us and we feel uplifted.

Finally, at the level of the Self, there is the G-Statement. While a B-Statement is uplifting in the moment, a G-Statement comes from the eternal truth. As we saw in Lecture 3, these are the wisdom statements found in every path and they bring us in touch with Shakti and divine Consciousness. They bring about spiritual peace.

The *Yoga Vashishta* suggests:

> O Rama, if you thus overcome this sorrow of repetitive history (*samsara*), you will live here on earth itself like a god, Brahma or Vishnu! For when delusion is gone and the truth is realised by means of inquiry into self-nature, when the mind is at peace and the heart leaps to the supreme truth, when all the disturbing thought-waves in the mind-stuff have subsided and there is unbroken flow of peace and the heart is filled with the bliss of the Absolute, when thus the truth has been seen in the heart, then this very world becomes an abode of bliss.

Each of these levels implies a different range of feeling and different understandings. In Self-inquiry, these levels are mountains we climb, being aware of the shifts in feeling and understanding as we travel on.

Let's see what actually happens during a session of group-inquiry.

THE STEPS OF GROUP-INQUIRY

1. Guided meditation

2. Giving the report

3. Deciding who should play

4. First player's statement and questions on story

5. Feedback—A-Statements

6. Checking feedback

7. Giving B- (and G-) Statements

8. D-Statements

9. Successive players.

1. GUIDED MEDITATION

In the Shiva Process inquiry group, participants sit in a circle. The form of the circle is historically a symbol of divine perfection and oneness. As the participants turn their awareness to the centre of the circle, they echo the Shaivite teaching that the Absolute is both *prakasha*, shining light, and *vimarsha*, Self-reflection.

In the late '80s, I did some work with Richard Monka's Ark Institute in Los Angeles. Monka used a group process which—though very different from my old ideas—reawakened something in me. I observed how powerful the experience of sitting in a circle was. *Vimarsha*, the capacity of *prakasha* to be aware of itself, includes language ability. In the circle, each person shines with the light of awareness. Rather than merely having a conversation, could we use the different perspectives represented by each individual as a self-reflecting mirror? The key to this was the discovery of a method of feedback.

The inquiry begins with a guided meditation. The leader asks the group to reflect on four chakras—the navel, heart, throat and third eye—and discover the feeling in each. The leader then asks participants to silently determine the best (most comfortable) chakra and also the worst. That done, everyone reports, moving clockwise, on what they have discovered. In all rituals in India, everything is done clockwise, and group-inquiry is ritual in the highest sense.

When you first go to a holy site, you walk around it once or three times, always moving clockwise. That is considered the 'right-hand path'. If you go the opposite way, then you are probably dabbling in the dark arts. If you want to practise the dark arts, then do everything anticlockwise: say the mantra with your *mala* (rosary) in your left hand. I am sure that you will get great powers of mind. Unfortunately, horrible things might happen to you as a consequence.

2. GIVING THE REPORT

Going around the room, every participant gives their report based on the guided meditation. One person says, for example, 'I felt a contraction in my navel'. Another might say, 'My navel was good, but I felt fear in my heart'. A third might say, 'All my chakras are relaxed and comfortable'. A fourth says, perhaps, 'I feel anger in my navel and sadness in my heart'.

3. DECIDING WHO SHOULD PLAY

Having heard all the reports, the leader, maybe in consultation with the group, decides who should 'play'. Notice the word 'play'. Ma Devi tells me that the term used in Gestalt is 'work', as in, 'Who is going to work now?' In the spirit of Shaivism, I prefer the word 'play' for the Shiva Process group. The sages speak of the 'sport' of Shiva, the *lila* of Shiva. Holding it that way gives a lightness to our enterprise, even though it is quite serious.

The decision about who should play first is intuitive. The leader might look for where the biggest block is. That might determine the person who most *needs* to play. Or the leader might look for the one who is most ready to play, who is practically spilling into the centre. Or the player who seems most interesting, whose play would be the most fun, might be chosen. When I lead a group, I sometimes ask three people to each name three people who are candidates to play. Where they agree is where we usually begin. The general rule, however, is to first go where the biggest block is.

This is a different spiritual method from *satsang*. In *satsang*, you don't pay attention to the blocks. In *satsang*, you always relate to the highest truth. Those who are open and can get in touch with it are uplifted, but the ones who are blocked suffer intensely. The Shakti increases their suffering as it hits against their blocks. Then they either experience a breakthrough or get more and more contracted. Thus, while *satsang* looks for upliftment and ignores blocks, Shiva Process looks to unblock them. The Shiva Process is compassionate. It asks, 'Who is hurting?' *Satsang*, on the contrary, says, 'Let them be uplifted or let them die at the side of the road'. In the Shiva Process we take the wounded and we carry them. I am not impugning *satsang*. Nothing is greater than true *satsang*, which evokes the divine presence. I'm simply saying that the inquiry group is a different method.

When Baba Muktananda transformed my understanding by telling me to always think, 'I am Shiva. I am neither a king nor a beggar', he was pointing me to the divine core that is within every person. Yogis identify with that core and not with their personal dramas. In the same way, group-inquiry comes from the perspective 'You are Shiva'. You are not neurotic, hung up or a sinner. It focuses on the energy of the higher Self and teaches every participant to access it. You may have blocks in various aspects of your life, but a new understanding can remove them.

The underlying faith of Shiva Process group-inquiry is that a new understanding is always available to free you, although it may be hidden. The method of group process is designed to discover that understanding. As a fall-back position, the A-Statement is always available: 'I am blocked at work' or 'I am blocked with my parents' and so on. The A-Statement acknowledges that there are moments when our yogic resources are not adequate to reach the truth, and there are times when one's best effort is to surrender to that uncertainty.

4. FIRST PLAYER'S STATEMENT AND QUESTIONS ON STORY

Now a player has been selected. The player is asked to describe their present state ('I feel ...') and concisely include a bit of story relevant to their feeling: something that happened in the office, something that happened at home, and so on. The leader asks the group, 'Are there any questions?' Here, the leader means questions about the story. The questions will be about events in space and time, not about feeling. What happened? Who said what? The story, you could say, is the personal part, the human part. I've been emphasising that the story is secondary to the awareness of the movement of Consciousness, but, nonetheless, it has a role.

DIVINE SHIVA PROCESS: GROUP-INQUIRY WITHOUT STORY

While the yogi in us may want to resolve everything into Consciousness, story is allowed its place as a way of honouring the personal element. It is also possible to do what I call a *Divine Shiva Process*, where you eliminate story completely. This is sometimes useful when the story element can't be brought out for reasons of privacy or when the player cannot make a connection between feeling and story. For example, the player says, 'I am angry'. In normal group-inquiry we say, 'When did you get angry, what happened?' The player says,

'Well, today something happened'. But in Divine Shiva Process, we don't ask that question. The player says, 'I am angry' and the group investigates that feeling of anger in the moment, unrelated to any story. Anger's causes probably lie deeper than the player knows anyway. Maybe something happened to them in early childhood, maybe in a past life. In the Divine Shiva Process, we don't go in search of those causes, but treat the anger as a sensation or entity in itself. Where is it? What does it feel like? How big is the feeling? What colour is it? In this way, you work with the feeling itself without seeking its causes. The technique of the Divine Shiva Process is related to *shambhavopaya*, the Shaivite method that ignores language and works directly with awareness.

A second version of the Divine Shiva Process is less austere. It allows feeling to reveal story, but the story is always about the player's relation to God or Self. I learned this method from my favourite 16th-century poet-saint Tukaram Maharaj. Tuka was a major Peculiar and he was always moving from one feeling to another. His genius was that he used every feeling as part of his relationship to God. He made it part of his drama or dialogue with the Divine. Applying this, if a player is angry, they might be angry at God or angry because they feel far from God. When Tuka felt weak, he would beg God for support. When Tuka felt strong, he would brag about his relationship with God. Let's get a sense of the Divine Shiva Process of this second kind.

INQUIRY: DIVINE SHIVA PROCESS

Look inside and see if there is a block in one of your centres. If there is not a block, then—hallelujah—just sit happily. If you feel there is a block (it might be in the navel or the heart or so on) then ask yourself, 'What is this about?' Your inner being will now throw up a story or a possibility: something happened today, or long ago or recently. The story comes up as one explanation. But in the Divine Shiva Process, we don't do that. Instead, we take the attitude: 'This block is about my relationship with God. This block is about my relationship with the Self.' Looking at it that way, what is your interpretation? Give it that interpretation.

Let's open our eyes. What was your experience? [Audience member: 'I felt a constriction in my navel and I saw it was sadness that related to something that happened today. Instead of thinking of it in those terms, I thought of it as having to do with my relationship with God. So I thought, "I'm sad because I am not in relationship with divine love".'] Yes, very good. Even though your feeling can be traced to a mundane experience, a mundane cause, it can also be framed in terms of your relationship with the Self or the Divine.

[Another audience member: 'I felt a block in my navel, which revealed itself as intolerance. Then I applied that to my relationship with God and I saw that my intolerance separates me from God.'] Good. You saw you had a choice not to be intolerant, and that being intolerant blocked you. That's good—that's applying real wisdom power to your situation.

Another way you could work with intolerance is to say, 'I am intolerant of my limitations'—there are a number of ways to go with it. This is the Divine Shiva Process. I recommend you use it on yourself. You can always describe anything in terms of your relationship with God. From one perspective, that is all that is going on, always. We think it is about this person or that person, but it is all about our relationship with Consciousness, with Self.

5. FEEDBACK–A-STATEMENTS

> There's a part of ourselves we can never know, so the world is set up as a reflection of ourselves in other people.
>
> **Ma Devi**

After the player's statement and the questioning that may be used to draw out the story comes a unique and essential feature: feedback. Feedback, as it used in group-inquiry, is the very heart of the method. Here the listeners reflect to the player what they have heard and experienced. Shiva Process is a discipline and a ritual. There is disciplined speaking and empathic listening. It teaches us to listen openly and on many levels. You hear what the player says literally, and you also try to hear into the meaning and feeling behind the words. Then you give feedback.

You ask yourself, 'What is the player actually saying or expressing?' When you get an internal answer, you give it as feedback. You say aloud, 'I am [the player's name] and I feel ...' You offer A-Statements to the player that reflect their state to them, *as you see or feel it*, after you listen to the player.

You will notice that the convention we use is to give the player's name when giving feedback to emphasise that you are mirroring the player's point of view. Now the player repeats the feedback statement with eyes closed, examining its effect on the inner world. The player repeats it as given, including their name. The effect of that is to create more detachment.

For example, Chuck is playing. Alfonse says, 'I'm Chuck and I feel angry'. Chuck repeats, 'I'm Chuck and I feel angry'. Lisa says, 'I'm Chuck and I feel disappointed'. Chuck repeats, 'I'm Chuck and I feel disappointed'. Chuck will not comment on the feedback (whether it's accurate or not), but simply observe how it fits or affects his inner world when he repeats it.

One way of finding the feedback you want to give to a player is to see what arises in *you* as you listen to the player. Then give it as feedback. When you give feedback, you don't have to worry if it is accurate or not, or whether it actually applies to the other person or not. You can simply give it, allowing the player to determine which statements are accurate and which are not. Sometimes a person intentionally gives inaccurate feedback to define an area of inquiry. This is not done indiscriminately, but may be used when a polarity statement clarifies where the player is at or, more precisely, is not at. Ultimately, only the player is the final judge of what is happening in their inner world.

Feedback is strong medicine. Consciousness is a luminous mirror. You look into that mirror when you engage in group-inquiry. You stare into the mirror of Consciousness, the mirror of your Self. I have said that there is one subject and many objects, but that other people are a special kind of object because they are subjects in their own right. When you sit facing other people, you are facing other conscious subjects, other Shivas. When you sit with them, you may be blind to your own unconscious, but they are not.

Don't you know things about your friends they don't know about themselves? Take that one step further and apply it to yourself. It bears repeating: even if you are blind to your own unconscious, others are not. That is true in life in general and in group-inquiry in particular. For a paranoid person, it is a nightmare that others know parts of their unconscious that are hidden to them, but that is the case. In group-inquiry, we recognise that by illuminating our unconscious to each other, we help each other.

The unconscious is simply those areas of the inner world that we don't see or don't want to see. Each of us is deeply involved in personal success and failure and how we appear to other people. But the person next to you is not concerned with you in that way at all. They don't care whether you look good or not. Au contraire! But to you, it is life and death. Because of their detachment from your attachment, they can give you information, but it should be done with compassion and empathy.

An individual ego is one point of view out of infinite points of view that actually or possibly exist in the universe. Ego is not simply a point of view, but it is also charged with emotion. It is deeply invested in outcomes and preferences. On the other hand, divine Consciousness includes all points of view at once. It does not worry about the individual ego at all—in fact, it crushes ego and grinds it underfoot. It does not heed our pleas for this, that and the other thing. Of course, I am dramatising this a bit, because divine Consciousness also includes compassion.

Group-inquiry replicates divine Consciousness by presenting a multiplicity of points of view. Mystically, the group as a whole speaks for the Divine. As individuals we are egos, but as a collective we reflect divinity. But even if, as I am saying, the voice of the group (when it is truly heard) reflects the voice of God, participants sometimes do not accept it as such. They sense a conspiracy—everyone is ganging up. In fact, such collusions rarely, if ever, occur. In general, players receiving feedback get an accurate snapshot of their unconscious. There are safeguards against victimising an individual, and in my experience, the groups have a lot of goodwill. The feedback one gets is valuable and worth heeding.

Normal life is no different. Life is simply a larger group process. Life also gives us accurate feedback, but we don't listen. Group process is highly clarified, a laboratory situation, but it is not a different reality. In this, it is like an ashram. A true ashram is a mysterious place in which feedback comes intensely, but the same truth exists outside the ashram and the same principles hold sway.

Other people's opinions of us, their thoughts about us, can be most terrifying. If we have a paranoid streak, then we are always worrying about what other people think of us and imputing all kinds of hateful thoughts to them. Now, here in group process, we're asked not to fear other people, but to see them as having goodwill and not enmity towards us—and to embrace their feedback as our most valuable ally. This is a real turning around of our normal perspective and immediately transforms our universe.

Nonetheless, we should be aware that feedback can sometimes be contaminated. There is good and there is bad feedback. Let's say Devadatta is playing and we give him feedback in the form, 'I'm Devadatta and I feel angry. I'm Devadatta and I feel hurt'. That's fine. But if I am angry at Devadatta and I say to Devadatta, 'I am Devadatta and I am disgusting'—that is bad feedback! It would be *good* feedback if Devadatta were actually saying to himself, 'I am a disgusting person'—then it would be accurate. But if it is judgment posing as feedback then it is really bad. And, unfortunately, that does happen.

Again, I may have a negative reaction to Devadatta and come up with the feedback, 'I am Devadatta and I am full of ego'. Nobody says within, 'I am full of ego'. That is not the way it comes from inside. A statement like that is a judgment that one person makes of another. However, in the world and in life, you are going to get feedback of that kind, and you are going to have to separate it from real feedback. Real feedback occurs when you tune into another; when you walk in another's shoes. It is empathic. When it is pure, it comes from the player and not from the feedback giver. It is a selfless act.

RIGHT SPEECH

In this way, group-inquiry puts a discipline on speech. Everywhere in life, undisciplined speech creates conflict and suffering.

One form of undisciplined speech is anger 'dumping'. Here, you take your anger accrued in one circumstance and indiscriminately spread it round elsewhere, creating sticky webs of karma that aren't easy to clean up. Another form of undisciplined speech is a phenomenon I call 'talking yourself down'. I am thinking of one person in my early life who used to begin speaking in a good mood and by the end of a few sentences was in misery. Nothing had happened. It was just the flow of her own *matrika* that brought her down. Some people do that a lot—in the process of speaking, they make themselves more depressed.

Scripture says that speech should be uplifting. In practice, it is often not that way. I grew up in New York, and negative speech was part of that culture: complaining, or attacking somebody behind their back. That culture of negative speech became an ingrained habit. In group-inquiry, such undiscriminating speech sticks out like a sore thumb and, usually, gets cleaned up at once.

The path of yoga, as well as the Buddha's eightfold path, is closely linked to understanding *matrika*. Thought-forms, whether in the mind or expressed through speech, should be uplifting and create an upward shift. When the Buddha refers to right speech, that is what he means. Hence, a yogi has to eliminate downward-tending patterns like complaining, negativity and fault-finding, and, inwardly, tearing thoughts.

Swami Muktananda says:

> What's the point of thinking about others? What's the point of finding fault with others? Once you begin to find fault with others, those faults get reflected in you, and there is no point in that. If you can restrain these negative vibrations, you will find only nectar, pure nectar flowing within. If you can do that you will overcome all your physical and mental ailments.

6. CHECKING FEEDBACK

Finally, we ask the player, 'Do any of the feedback statements you've received resonate with you? Do you like any of them?' *You* are the arbiter of what is happening inside of you. *Only you.* Your inner space is sacred and inviolate. No matter how intuitive other people may be, they are always external with regard to your inner space. Well, perhaps an enlightened being has merged with the universal 'I'. But even in the face of such a one, it is your own space and you have the right to say what is going on in there. Of course, you may be confused, or you may lie or be in denial.

For some people, receiving feedback can be daunting at first. They might feel they are being judged. They might be surprised at the accuracy of the statements. They often are inclined to comment, to reject certain statements as inaccurate, or they may temporarily fall deeper into tearing thoughts. But if they stay open and follow the process, statements will resonate.

After a number of A-Statements have been given, the leader must find out what the effect on the player has been, perhaps asking, 'Did you have a shift? Which statement caused the shift? Did any of them seem true? If so, which ones?' When the group is satisfied that the function of the A-Statements has been performed; that is, that the player has arrived at a clear and accurate description of their present feeling, then the leader calls for B-Statements, unless a shift has already happened. In that case, the leader should move on to a new player.

A shift is when the feeling moves from negative to positive or when a block is removed. It can be subtle, such as tension in the navel chakra dissolving or the heart chakra opening or a feeling of peace. It can also be more intense, marked by tears, laughter or understanding. In general, it is important to move on once a shift occurs, wherever it occurs in the process. This keeps the focus on Consciousness and not personal drama, and also prevents the group losing what it has gained.

'FIXING' PEOPLE

Because the Shiva Process emphasises the movement of Consciousness, its goal is to unblock awareness and not 'fix' people. That's why I encourage group leaders to move on to another player once a shift has occurred. This is the principle of small gains. The temptation is strong to continue processing the original player; that would indeed happen in story-oriented psychological groups. The faith of the Shiva Process is different, however. It says that if the group continually works to unblock awareness, everything is served; that this method is for the highest good of all participants.

While this is a simple protocol, in practice, it's hard to resist the temptation to overcook the process. When the discipline 'once a shift happens, move on' is not observed, the player tends to go back into their story and the feeling usually goes down. I believe if we serve the process properly, the optimum amount of 'fixing' actually takes place.

Perhaps the purest form of group-inquiry pays no attention to story, but only to the shifts of energy, as in the Divine Shiva Process. But it is good not to be fanatical about this, and to be tolerant of people's desire to solve problems. Nonetheless, our primary focus is always on the movement of energy.

7. GIVING B- (AND G-) STATEMENTS

The B-Statement is not feedback in the same way that the A-Statement is feedback. B-Statements do not come solely from the group's perception of the player; rather, they express the goodwill of the group towards the player, and are an offering.

When do we offer B-Statements? [Audience: 'After A-Statements!'] The completely correct answer is that you give B-Statements when it is time for B-Statements. That is the Zen answer. You just know. When you feel that the appropriate A-Statement has been said—when the player says, for example, 'I feel hurt' and the group is satisfied that it is the core statement of present feeling in the moment—then we go on. The A-Statement has located where the player is, and now B-Statements are given to help the person move towards the Self.

An A-Statement is powerful. It can create upliftment, and when it does, you might want to move on to the next player, even without going to B-Statements. In this case, you could say the A-Statement has acted as a B-Statement. Simply bearing witness to the truth in the form of an A-Statement can so please Consciousness that it creates an upward shift.

The A-Statement is like a homeopathic remedy in which you treat 'like with like'. The B-Statement is allopathic in that you treat something with its opposite. Patanjali, in a memorable aphorism, says, 'When the mind is troubled by negative thoughts, contemplate the opposite'. Thus, if you are filled with hatred, you should think about love; if you are filled with agitation, you should contemplate peace; if you are filled with sadness, you should think about a joyful memory.

Sometimes, a feedback statement, either an A- or B-Statement, has an unexpectedly powerful effect. We call such a statement a 'zinger'. It comes from left field, as it were, and captures the conscious mind by surprise, shocking it into sudden revelation. I suppose the ultimate zinger was God's 'Let there be light'. That caused a big shift and all kinds of havoc in its wake!

As I've said, G-Statements, scriptural statements, are a subset of B-Statements. They are particularly powerful because of their divine origin. G-Statements can be salted among the B-Statements or come at the end of B-Statements.

In the medical profession, there is some controversy about the merits of treating 'like with like' or 'like with unlike', but the universe seems to support both methods. I've already emphasised that it is good to make use of humanity's full wealth of G-Statements and not be limited to a particular path or religion. Hence it is not unusual to hear G-Statements from different traditions existing side by side during feedback: 'I'm X and Jesus loves me. I'm X and everything is Consciousness. I'm X and my self is an illusion. I'm X and I am the Self.' The Shiva Process is results-oriented. Like a doctor who is well versed in many modalities, and who uses both Western and Eastern medicine, the Shiva Process says, 'whatever works'.

THE QUESTION OF ADVICE

The impulse to give advice to a struggling friend is natural and compassionate. I see a person in trouble in a circumstance that I feel I understand and know how to master, and out of sympathy I offer my guidance. Advice implicitly says that if I were in your shoes, I would do it this way. When we're stuck, we get assailed by doubt and negative emotion. We don't see things clearly. Another person who is detached sees more clearly and wants to offer advice. Good counsel is valuable but infrequently followed. The receiver of guidance, already struggling with knowing what is the right or wrong course of action, has to be convinced it is good advice.

The best kind of advice comes about when it is asked for, not when the advice-giver is being a 'know-it-all'. Thus, in group-inquiry a rule has evolved: 'No unsolicited advice.' If a person wants to give a suggestion, they should say, 'I have advice, do you want to hear it?' and the player can agree to hear it or not.

When players receive feedback, it performs the same function as advice, only more powerfully. Through feedback they receive, as it were, their own advice. To validate the valuable place of guidance, the Shiva Process includes the *D-Statement* (action statement—see below).

When the impulse to give advice arises strongly in a group, it suggests that the player is extremely disempowered and out of touch with their wisdom voice. It may indicate that it's time to give D-Statements. Also, it might be that A-Statements like 'I feel disempowered. I feel uncertain. I feel lost' would be more useful, since the player is too disempowered to act on good advice anyway.

Once, feeling that the group was overflowing with advice it wanted to give to a player, I gave the following quirky but quintessentially Shiva Process contemplation. I told the player that he should open inwardly and that the other members of the group should silently send him advice. In the act of opening, he was able to 'hear' some of the guidance that was sent to him.

8. D-STATEMENTS

For the Shiva Process to be complete, there has to be a 'doing' that flows out of the thinking and feeling components. We exist not only in emotional and intellectual bodies, but also in the physical body. The three personality types, Peculiar, Solid and Vital, reflect the three energies of Kashmir Shaivism, *iccha*, *jnana* and *kriya*. Accordingly, after B- and G-Statements are given, the leader may call for D-Statements; that is, 'doing statements' or 'homework'. The leader can move to D-Statements by asking, 'What do you think you can do about that?' or

'How can you shift that?' After the player considers this for a while and makes suggestions, the group can then give D-Statements, some of which might not have occurred to the player.

The player resolves to put insights into action. The *Bhagavad Gita* says, 'Yoga is skill in action'. When we act on our insights, they become real in our lives. A D-Statement might be, 'I resolve to write my mother a letter' or 'I agree to clean up my room' or 'I will meditate every day this week' or 'I will speak to my boss about my issue'. Thus, action statements are given in the form of D-Statements rather than advice, and through these statements the group searches for the upward shift. A D-Statement is truly an 'offering' because the player decides which of them to adopt.

The three personality types, Solid, Vital and Peculiar, are reflected in the A-, B-, G- and D-Statements. The A-Statement represents the Solid. It is a cool, accurate and no-nonsense reflection of what is so. The B- and G-Statements represent the Peculiar. They are imaginative, upward aspirations of the soul. They give new and expansive possibilities. And finally, the D-Statement represents the Vital, acknowledging that thoughts and feelings must be expressed in action. In this way, the Shiva Process method includes all aspects of the three-tiered human animal.

Now that we've seen the whole movement of a group, we can refine our definition of the upward shift. It can be in one of three forms: feeling, thinking and doing. If the player has a release of feeling or tension, the group can move on. If the player has an important insight, the group can move on. If the player firmly resolves on a strong and specific course of action, the group can move on. Any of these constitute an upward shift, broadly defined. So, an upward shift galvanises a dormant or blocked Peculiar, Solid or Vital.

9. SUCCESSIVE PLAYERS

In group-inquiry, once the B-, G- and D-Statements are given, that person has finished playing and we move on to the next player. It's hoped the player has had an upward shift and the force of Consciousness has increased. The shape of a perfect Shiva Process group is that it begins in separation and contraction and, through brilliant work, the energy is uplifted, builds and gets higher, until all are ecstatic at the end. That's a perfect 10. But we don't always get there. Of course, sometimes we do.

When we don't, it is because our wisdom, insight, technique and many other factors are not, on this occasion, equal to the task of attaining divine awareness. And that should be okay for us, because what is important is the intention and the effort—the goodwill. Even in the worst case, inquiry is always interesting and always different. When you are talking about Consciousness, you are talking about something that is full of mystery and full of surprises. That's why I like to say that we can never *master* the Shiva Process, but rather we should think of ourselves as servants of the process.

I think that a few centuries from now, people will look back at our 21st-century methods of communication and regard them as extremely primitive and brutal, just as we look back, with superior amusement, on the scientific beliefs of a thousand years ago.

In our time, it is normal for people to throw negativity around indiscriminately and to speak and act out of unprocessed emotion. Through lack of inquiry and self-examination, they plunge their lives into darkness and confusion. In the future, inquiry will raise awareness significantly. People will become increasingly aware of the subtle dimensions of communication and thereby avoid a lot of suffering. They will look back on us in amazement that we could have lived so primitively.

SHIFTING STATEMENTS

I thought about reproducing a transcript of part of a group to provide a taste of actual group process. But a transcript doesn't do justice to the dynamism of what occurs. Then I remembered that for a number of years I collected significant *shifting statements*—statements that cause a shift—after each group. What follows is a selection from our files. They are A-, B-, G- and D-Statements. I haven't categorised them here, but what they have in common is that each of them had a powerful impact and even culminated the participant's play. Reading through these statements, I think, gives more of an idea of the true group process than would a transcript.

We used to collect all the statements of a participant and give them a print-out on their birthday. They could see the shape of their spiritual year and what had changed and what hadn't. Every statement suggests a story, they are like moments in a larger narrative. They provide flashes of insight into the human condition. Like the Sistine ceiling, where God and Adam almost touch fingers, they indicate a movement towards connection between the human and the Divine. As I reread them, I hear them as scripture, as sutras.

Here are some actual examples of shifting statements from our notebooks:

Please don't judge me.

Please be kind to me.

I'm yearning for love.

I'm attached to the game.

I have no time for my heart.

I'm full of blocked feeling.

Everything's going to be okay.

I live for love.

I will be fearless.

I feel free.

My deepest nature is a spiritual being.

God, help me break the cycle.

I love the Self.

I'm tearing into myself.

Please understand me.

I trust the flow of life.

All joy is Shiva. All suffering is Shiva.

Everyone has their dharma which can be discovered and expressed.

My heart is strong.

Nothing external can take away my bliss.

Being in a relationship won't change my feelings about myself.

I trust my feelings.

I will discipline my speech.

God is taking care of me.

I want to live in the present all the time.

Meditate first thing.

No drinking.

Do one stupid thing a day.

I will never get more than I can cope with.

I'm on the verge of a breakthrough.

Make only uplifting statements.

Spend time alone.

I surrender to God's will.

I can shift the feelings without changing outer circumstances.

I want God to be my boss.

Prayer is an empowered form of worry.

I let the past go.

I'm seeing more than I'm saying.

Be true to myself.

Get rid of tearing thoughts.

I want to know who I am.

I want to serve.

I want your attention, God.

GROUP-INQUIRY AND THERAPY

Because people sit in a circle and speak with each other about their inner world in group-inquiry, it might be mistaken for therapy. Unlike therapy, however, group-inquiry is not about 'opening up' but about expanding and following the Shakti. It is about the removal of blocks while paying keen attention to the spiritual energy. It gives understanding of how spiritual energy works, and teaches participants how to increase it. If we can't do that, at least we should begin to understand it.

From the highest point of view, the whole universe is engaged in inquiry. The universe is nothing but Consciousness discovering Itself. In the desert, the rocks sit and do the silent rock-like group-inquiry with each other. For some groups, therapy is the level of group-inquiry that is right and appropriate. But therapy is more interested in the drama of the personal than in the understanding of Consciousness. Sessions of chanting are a kind of group-inquiry in which the technique is simply to sing G-Statements. Shiva Process group-inquiry includes both the personal and impersonal, paying particular attention to the movement of Consciousness.

While therapy is concerned with helping a person get rid of neurosis and make a better adjustment to life, yoga seeks mystical oneness with the Divine. It seeks not adjustment, but Self-realisation. Surely, it would not be surprising if, as one practises yoga, one becomes less neurotic and more competent in many areas of life. The greater quest contains the lesser. Group-inquiry is a form of yoga: specifically, the yoga of wisdom.

In a therapy group, the focus is on the people in the group. In group-inquiry, the real focus is on the *space* at the centre of the group. That space is pure Consciousness and represents the relationship or *satsang* of everyone in that moment. That space can be pure and expansive or contaminated and contracted. It is as though the players build a mandala of feeling together, with the aim of expanding and purifying that feeling. The feeling in the group is never one person's problem or one person's fault, but everyone's joint koan.

Group-inquiry allows us to have the experience of sharing our inner world with others and working together with others to uplift that inner world. Shiva Process group work is as close to entering the mystery of another's subjectivity as is humanly possible, short of occult means. And occult means are notoriously spotty and haphazard, while the Shiva Process is dependable and repeatable. It is a unique experience. You learn to participate in another's inner world without getting personally caught up. Normal relationships always have the possibility of confusion. Group-inquiry has more objectivity.

In the same way, a relationship consists of two people, but the space between two people represents the relationship itself. On the day of a wedding, that relationship is filled with love and surrender. But as time goes on, different thoughts and feelings enter that space. When the space becomes contaminated by blame and recrimination, the relationship suffers. A marriage relationship is a group-inquiry for two. When the couple understands how to follow the upward shift and eliminate blocks, the relationship is strong and nurturing.

When I say the group creates a mandala of feeling, I am referring to the sand mandalas that certain Tibetan Buddhist monks create. They painstakingly, over several days, create a beautiful multicoloured pattern from coloured sand. It becomes a container of subtle energy. At the end, the mandala is simply destroyed. At the end of each inquiry group, the mandala of feeling is also uncreated. The important thing is not to build something permanent, but to build and rebuild the mandala—watching the movement of Consciousness. In the case of Self-inquiry groups, not every mandala is beautiful. In the best of all possible worlds, each group would be a steady triumph over ignorance, ending in a mutual experience of the Divine. Sometimes our skill is not up to that, but the process is always worthwhile and revealing.

EXPANSION OF CONSCIOUSNESS

In group-inquiry, we have to keep our focus on two things at once: story and the movement of Consciousness. As I've mentioned, group-inquiry is spirituality, not therapy, yet it includes therapy. You could think of Shiva Process group-inquiry as worship of Consciousness, the study of Consciousness, or even the ritual purification of Consciousness. It involves observing the play of *matrika* against the background of feeling, and watching for shifts.

What is really interesting is the movement of upward and downward shifts. Spiritually considered, the key moments in your life are the moments when you contract and expand. There are always reasons for these movements and they are always revealing. In group-inquiry, we watch those contractions and expansions carefully. You see, for example, how tearing thoughts bring you down, and how G-Statements, when they work well, uplift you. You can observe all of this directly and clearly.

Usually, each of us lives in a fairly well-defined mental world. We move rather mechanically amid a familiar range of thoughts and feelings, whether these come from our childhood training or are somehow intrinsic to us. Sometimes we feel our inner space to be constricted or boring, whereas, in the process of receiving feedback, we draw on funds of *matrikas* from other people. We borrow other people's minds and points of view, which allow us to think 'outside the box'. The 'box' is our habitual mind with grooves formed by repetitive patterns of thinking and feeling, and this creates a closed structure. If we stay inside that structure, we stay inside the normal pattern of our suffering.

Even though other minds may be in their own boxes, they are outside your particular box and can help you to see things in a new way. Feedback from others' minds quite literally expands ours, lifts us out of mechanical patterns and gives us new inspiration. We are each outside the box to each other and can perform this service for each other.

The mind's box is its arena of conscious thoughts. Outside the box is the unconscious. When our minds open, the unconscious becomes conscious and our whole being takes a breath. G-Statements, scripture and the teachings of the sages work the same way as feedback, by bringing in new possibilities, creating greater interior spaciousness and expanding the mind.

QUESTIONS AND ANSWERS

FEELING LOST

Question: Sometimes I feel lost in a group and I don't know where it's going, and this is sometimes true of personal inquiry, too.

Swamiji: This is a mysterious world, isn't it? Don't you find it so? Wouldn't it be surprising if as soon as you started doing inquiry you had complete clarity? But inquiry goes through many different terrains. Some of them are difficult, unpleasant and confusing. When that happens, I take refuge in the A-Statement and an all-purpose question I have for myself. Shall I tell you this secret or make you shovel buffalo dung for 12 years?

Oh, all right, the question I ask myself is 'How can I get as close as possible to what's so?' Isn't this the essence of inquiry, to focus on what's real and present? The answer to that question will be an A-Statement: 'I feel confused' or 'I feel lost' or 'I feel tense.' Such an A-Statement puts you on track in terms of your inquiry.

DISCIPLINING ANGER

Question: Sometimes in Shiva Process groups I've been in, people use feedback as an opportunity to vent anger at the person playing. Could you comment on this?

Swamiji: Yes, this does happen. Someone in the group has a reaction to the player—they get angry because one of their own issues is activated, or they become judgmental if they perceive dishonesty. I certainly don't have to enumerate all the reasons people get angry. Experience shows that anger has to submit to a strong discipline. In the early days of group-inquiry, anger was bandied about in ways that turned out to be destructive. People sometimes left the group feeling wounded. If a strong reaction of this kind comes up, it indicates the play has shifted from the original player to the reactant person. The anger that has arisen has to go back inside the second person and be processed there. In other words, the angry person should become the player. Feeling moves around the group from player to player and determines who is to play.

Anger enlivens a group, but in an unpleasant way. When anger enters, people become intensely present because there is danger in the air. As I've mentioned, in the early days of our group work, some people were addicted to the thrill of anger in the group. Anger can signify there is a lot of *truth* and little *kindness*. The opposite situation, when kindness is excessive and eliminates truth, creates a condition of safety, but a dead and boring kind of safety. Think of the atmosphere of a cocktail party (I'm thinking of the faculty parties I used to go to when I couldn't avoid them): everyone is being polite and politically correct and danger is absent, but transformation is not happening. As I have said many times, things are really happening in a group when there is truth and kindness in equal measure.

Regard the group as Shiva or universal Consciousness. While an individual may be 'off'—personal elements like anger or judgment distorting their view—the collective is generally not off. Of course, there can be groups that are completely wrong, like the collection of Nazis in Germany, but, in general, the group is a fairly accurate reflection of Shiva.

Wisdom does not reside solely in a particular person, however evolved. The wisdom resides in Shiva, and different people—all being Shiva—can manifest that wisdom at any moment. That is why they say *Siddhas*, realised beings, can learn from an idiot and teach the wise. They are open to God speaking through anyone, any time and in any place. So, in group-inquiry, that wisdom is contained in the sum total of all the individual awarenesses.

BALANCING TRUTH AND KINDNESS

Question: You mention that inquiry groups which have more truth than kindness tend to be exciting but frightening. On the other hand, groups that have more kindness than truth tend to feel safe but boring. Do you have any tips for attaining a balance?

Swamiji: In inquiry groups, the solution to a multitude of problems lies in being aware of what *is* in any moment and bearing witness to it. Say what is so. Once you acknowledge that a group is kindly but boring, you could say, 'This group needs more truth' or 'We're being too polite'. The group can make a decision to increase the truth factor. It will feel as though everyone has simultaneously awakened from a dream or a stupor.

It's never that inquiry fails us, it's rather that we fail inquiry. The Shiva Process hinges on what we bring to it. If we bring courage and aliveness and a resolve to get close to the truth, the process will hum.

These issues have general application in our lives as well. Some of us live our lives in a mediocre way, never stepping up to the bar. Others are always overstepping and getting burnt. You could do the following meditation, which will also help you in group work to learn how to intensify or relax the group as needed:

CONTEMPLATION: A HALF-STEP FORWARD OR BACK

- *Contemplate taking a half-step further into your life.* Imagine living your life just *slightly* more fully and honestly, and with more passion. This is an antidote to excessive kindness. You will increase the energy in your life. Don't let everything slide. Speak up. In your meditation, you can ask yourself, 'What would this or that aspect of my life be like if I took a half-step further into it?'

- *Take a half-step back from your life.* Imagine living your life with *slightly* more detachment. Don't take everything personally and emotionally. Don't react to every person and event. This is an antidote for too much engagement. In your meditation, you can imagine taking a philosophical view of things that occur, seeing everything as the will of God or the play of Consciousness.

THE ART OF LISTENING

Question: I've noticed that when some people play, I am riveted and hang on every word, while when others play, my mind wanders. Could you comment on this?

Swamiji: You've noticed an important thing. In some forms of group work, participants are taught the right way to 'listen'. They are encouraged to be open, silent, empathic and try to hear what is being said and listen also for deeper layers of what is being said. These are all good things, but you point out a real truth.

It is much easier to listen to someone who is in touch with the Self than to someone who is out of touch. If you find your mind wandering, it surely means that the person playing has not connected to the mother lode of energy, which the truth would yield. Your boredom and lack of concentration may indicate that more truth is necessary and that the group is being led down a false or at least not a fruitful path.

Alternatively, it could indicate that *you* should play! Another reason for your mind wandering is that you might have become unpresent. You may be thinking about other things. Or you may have a block; perhaps a fear of your own emotion. Maybe one of your issues has been triggered.

Dig deep in such cases and find a more accurate feedback. If you find it, it will bring more energy into the room. Remember this: Consciousness is listening, the room is listening, the true Self is listening. Your true Self always knows what's going on, even when your mind doesn't.

GIVING AND RECEIVING FEEDBACK

Question: I have trouble coming up with feedback during the process. Do you have any hints?

Swamiji: You are trying too hard to give perfect and accurate feedback. Just let fly. Feedback is something we offer, and the player decides to accept it or not, whether it is relevant or not. So don't be such a perfectionist. Feedback that is not true can be important because it shows the player where they are not, which is good information to have. It confirms, 'Oh no, that's not right'.

Consider paying less attention to your thoughts, and access your feeling in the moment, then offer it as feedback as though it were the player's feeling. You will be surprised how often that is the case.

Question: The first time I received feedback in the Shiva Process group, it was an astounding experience. I didn't know so much of me was visible! It wasn't frightening, but it was like being with intimates who loved and knew me even though I hadn't met them before. Could you say something more about feedback?

Swamiji: I agree with you, it's quite mind-boggling the first time you experience it. Feedback lies at the very heart of the Shiva Process. Through feedback, the unconscious becomes conscious. Good feedback demonstrates that people have been listening with empathy and attention, listening through their pores, not only with their ears.

One of the values implicit in the Shiva Process is that each participant is an important part of universal Consciousness. If that's true, it's highly desirable that people participate. I like to encourage everyone to give feedback. If I notice someone not giving feedback, I might pause and try to help that person find their feedback. You can find your feedback by paying attention to what you perceive in the other person, what you yourself are thinking, and what you are feeling.

I also encourage participants to pace their feedback so there's time for the player to absorb it. Sometimes there's a wealth of feedback that springs up, usually because the player has brought so much feeling into the room. The rest of the group may respond with 'machine-gun' feedback, one after another, sometimes with one person giving multiple feedback, which doesn't allow the player time to digest it.

Another important point about feedback—it is tremendous acknowledgment of another person. I remember a transformational group 30 years ago that discovered the importance of acknowledging others, hence its members used to run around saying, 'I really want to acknowledge you for that'. It was a bit obvious, but it still works, because people so love to be acknowledged. I think that when you get accurate feedback, it is supreme acknowledgment because it shows you've been heard and understood on a very deep level. Explicit acknowledgment is important, too. So in the closing questions, which we will explore in the following lecture, there's a section where people can acknowledge that session's star performers.

Question: Isn't receiving A-Statements as feedback a little bit like having a psychic reading?

Swamiji: Maybe it's a little bit like having a psychic reading, but there's an important distinction. When you go for a psychic reading, the psychic *tells* you what's going on in your inner space. In group-inquiry, the A-Statements are not a 'telling' but an 'offering'. My intention regarding the Shiva Process ethic is that only you are the ultimate judge of your own experience. You are the only person who inhabits your inner world and only you can ultimately say what's going on there. Sometimes a person is in denial about what's really going on or has pushed it into their unconscious, and therefore A-Statements are quite surprising and revealing. Nonetheless, it's up to you and you alone to say, 'That one was relevant. That one gave me a shift'.

Also, giving feedback is different from a psychic because there is no pressure on the feedback giver to be always right. Psychics sometimes develop an oracular quality because everything they say has to be authoritative. A feedback giver can relax and let fly. There's no problem if they are wrong because the validation will come from the player, the feedback receiver.

Having said that, one of the effects of doing a lot of group-inquiry is the development of psychic sensitivity. People develop the ability to 'tune in' to what others are saying, both at the level of text and subtext.

Question: When I've received feedback in groups, it makes me feel defensive. I want to reject most statements as they make me feel threatened.

Swamiji: I would urge you to respectfully entertain the feedback you are given. Feedback is a marvellous process. Sometimes you say something in a group and you get a whole wealth of feedback; it just *pours* out of everyone. If a lot of the feedback surprises you, it's really good! It means that your psyche has hidden things from yourself and now you will see them. When you hear something that seems odd to you, it is precisely then that you should pay particular attention. You may learn something about your unconscious. It is a great boon to see your unconscious. I became *insane* to see my unconscious at one stage of my *sadhana*—I was desperate to see it. It is like seeing the back of your head. The back of your head is obvious to everybody else, but not to you. Try turning your head really quickly and see if you can get a glimpse of it. I mean, the flowing locks on the back of my head are obvious to all of you, aren't they? In the same way, our unconscious is much more obvious to others than to ourselves. I love searching for the unconscious. Learn to relish it.

SHIVA PROCESS AND THERAPY

Question: I know you don't like comparisons of Shiva Process with psychology, but it does seem somewhat similar to cognitive psychology. Could you comment on that?

Swamiji: Yes, of course there are certain similarities. In cognitive psychology, the practitioner identifies debilitating thoughts, or tearing thoughts, classifies them and remoulds them to reflect a more balanced view. This achieves a shift in perspective which also brings about a shift in mood or feeling. There are differences as well, but if you think about it, it is not surprising that Shiva Process will share some similarities with any psychological process.

Shiva Process is simply the recognition of blocks, the freeing of those blocks, and the reinforcement of the flow precipitated by that release. As such, it is a universal template. Not only does cognitive psychology follow this pattern, but many religious rituals do as well.

At the heart of the Tibetan Buddhist *chod* practice is a visualisation whereby practitioners merge their consciousness with the Divine, then offer their inert body as a feast for the suffering beings ('demons' in Tibetan taxonomy; *matrikas* in Shiva Process) that create havoc in the lives of humans. The 'sacrifice' or 'cutting through' is an offering. It is made without defences. A few practitioners of *chod* have told me that the systems feel the same: the Shiva process play with its upward shift, and the visualised sacrifice of the *chod* with its satiation of the demons. Apparently, there are parallels in the *chod* system with the A-, B- and G-Statements. Again, isn't this universal spirituality? You begin in block or ignorance, and you work through it and open to grace or upliftment.

So, yes, there are similarities to cognitive therapy, but there are also differences. As far as I know, cognitive therapy is not aware of the Self or universal Consciousness, and is not aimed at Self-realisation. As a tool for making a person calmer and happier, however, it certainly has its place.

Question: Could you say something about the difference between group-inquiry and psychoanalysis?

Swamiji: I'd love to! Look, the ocean is very deep. It has many, many things hidden within it. If we explore the ocean, we can find some of them—childhood traumas, histories of abuse, even past-life tragedies. But, at any particular moment, only a few things are washed up on the beach. While psychoanalysis tends to plumb the depths of the ocean, in Shiva Process we examine what is thrown up on the beach, moment to moment. In other words, we have faith in the power of Consciousness as it manifests in the present moment. The present moment gives you what you need. Awareness is focused and most vivid in the present.

You shouldn't become dogmatic about this, however, because it can happen that the present moment may throw up a memory of a trauma, or even a rebirthing. Anything can be thrown up on that shore. It could be that you need to go through a memory of something that happened when you were three—that could come up. But to entertain the theory that you have to do that every time is not correct. You have to be open and alert. Everything is possible, but everything changes as well.

Question: I heard you mention that you're dubious about the question 'why?' and you prefer the question 'what?'

Swamiji: Why do you say that? No, it's true. I'm partial to the question 'What's going on here?' With 'what', we look at that which actually exists, while with 'why' there's always the danger of drifting off into mental realms or tearing thoughts. Salman Rushdie means something similar when he says that '"What if?" is an uninteresting question compared to "what is?"'. Therapy tends to ask 'why?' and spends a long time hunting for causes. My point of view is that there's direct information to be gained by dealing with the is-ness of things.

Take the case of Charlie Brown's famous quote as sung by The Coasters, 'Why's everybody always pickin' on me?' The answer to that question could be, 'Because you're a jerk, Charlie Brown' or because you're a Peculiar or because your mother didn't love you. I'd rather hear Charlie Brown make an A-Statement, 'People are always picking on me', and then go to a deeper level of truth by letting us know how he feels: 'I feel sad.' Now we're out of the area of tearing thoughts and speculation and into actuality. In future songs, Charlie Brown will emerge as an empowered and self-aware individual. Of course, the songs won't be as good.

ONE EYE IN, ONE EYE OUT

Question: What relationship does Self-inquiry have to meditation?

Swamiji: Self-inquiry can certainly be seen as a form of meditation. Ramana Maharshi made the distinction between meditation as it's normally understood—the use of an image, mantra or idea—and inquiry, which superimposes nothing but rather strips everything extraneous away.

I like to make the following distinction. In normal life, we keep both of our eyes open, paying attention to our environment and other people. In meditation, we shut both of our eyes and focus entirely on our inner world, dissolving all thoughts and memories of the outer world.

In Shiva Process inquiry, we keep one eye open and one eye closed; that is, by means of inquiry, we operate effectively in the outer world, never losing touch with the movement of the inner world. When people do group-inquiry, this double attention is perfected. They have to participate in what happens in the group while being particularly sensitive to subtle inner changes.

Self-inquiry of the Shiva Process type can be used in the world of form to solve human problems. This does not mean that it is limited to the realm of form, because effective inquiry will often dip into the transcendental state. In Shiva Process groups, there are, not infrequently, moments which are sometimes called *shambhavopaya* moments, where a thought-free state descends and a sense of oneness arises. If you want to distinguish Self-inquiry from other forms of meditation, the defining characteristic is that inquiry uses a questioning method to go deeper.

GROUP-INQUIRY WHEN YOU'RE FEELING GOOD

Question: Sometimes I find in the group that I feel really good and there are no contractions. Can I still play? Can you participate in group-inquiry when you're not feeling contracted?

Swamiji: When you feel that way, that is very good. You can help others undo their contractions. In other words, you can serve them. In this form of inquiry, we unblock blocks. It is a *via negativa*, we expel disease. We could do a process that moves towards feeling good and ignores the contraction. As I've said, that would be more like the method of *satsang*.

It is heroic and compassionate to risk your good state when you do this work, because when we link up in the group we intensely relate to everyone else there, and we can be brought down. An experienced Shiva Process person learns how to enter fully into that relationship and feel all the feelings and yet emerge unscathed, like a guitar string that vibrates a note for a while and then is still. You shouldn't be too concerned, as some participants are, of 'taking on' feelings from the group. When you participate in group work, you take a kind of *bodhisattva* vow; that is, a commitment not to become realised until all beings have done so. We're all part of the one universal Consciousness, so no one can really achieve individual salvation. Each person must try to uplift every other person. So, you have to get your hands dirty and work for the good of the whole.

The following are questions on A-, B- and G-Statements. As we've seen repeatedly, different kinds of statements contain different levels of energy and feeling. Tearing thoughts contain negative energy; A-Statements, a much more positive energy; and B- and G-Statements, usually an even more uplifting form of energy. A meditator tries to become a 'Lord of Matrika'; that is, tries to control self-talk. By cultivating positive self-talk, we transform the quality of our life and come closer to the Self.

B-STATEMENTS

Question: Sometimes when I make a B-Statement, it brings up a tearing thought. Do you have any suggestions?

Swamiji: One way to get around this is to use what I call subjunctive B-Statements. We used to use the grammatical term, 'condition contrary to fact'. So, instead of saying, 'I can meditate', which brings up a definite, 'No you cannot' from below, say instead, 'I wish I could meditate'. You will feel completely one with this statement and it may very well act as a B-Statement for you. Similarly, instead of saying, 'I still my mind', say, 'I wish my mind were still'. This is similar to my insight about having the meditation you are having. You may not be able to meditate, but you can certainly wish to meditate. You may not be able to still your mind, but you can certainly wish to still your mind. This understanding has wide applications. Self-acceptance is at the core of it. Always take refuge in getting as close as possible to what is so, and bearing witness to that.

Question: A B-Statement seems like an affirmation. Is there a difference?

Swamiji: To affirm and to inquire are two different processes. Both are human and both have their place. When we affirm something, we insist on a certain outcome and we affirm our particular answer. When we inquire, we ask a question and let an answer come to us. While the process of affirming is strong, there is also a danger in it. Affirmation can create ego inflation and 'wrong crystallisation', a situation in which spiritual growth increases ego rather than eliminates it. You have to ask what is under any particular affirmation—what voice, what force, what emotion lies beneath? Powerful figures throughout history, both religious and political, have strongly affirmed one thing or another and sometimes created great havoc. That's why science, for example, trusts only the process of inquiry and not affirmation. And Zen, too, trusts only inquiry.

You could ask, who has the right to affirm? Does an angry person, a vengeful person, a judgmental person, a self-righteous person? Many affirmations come from such a source. And the impurity of the source is communicated. Surely only Shiva or the Self has the right to affirm, because that is the space of pure love and pure awareness. Therefore, I think the proper order of things is to first inquire and only then affirm. Look within, see what lies underneath, find the pure space of the Self and then strongly make an affirmation from that position.

Question: Sometimes I find a B-Statement and it might give me an upward shift, but then I have a nagging thought that the B-Statement might not be true and I might be putting myself into a fool's paradise. What should I do?

Swamiji: This is a universal question and it has to do with truth and validation. In outer things, we validate our understandings by gathering evidence. When the evidence is strong enough, we say the thing is 'true'. Now, how do you validate either of these two statements: 'I am a loser' or 'I am Shiva'? You can muster evidence for being a loser, such as a pathetic past history, and this will spontaneously spring up when you are in a negative state. In this case, your evidence is impure because your depression, and not the facts, is speaking. For 'I am Shiva' you can muster evidence like 'Scripture tells me so. Shaivism says ... The Guru says ...' In this case, because you are quoting authoritative sources, there is validity.

However, the kind of validity I am speaking about is experiential or inner validity. When you experience a taste of the inner Self, you get an upward shift of some kind. From this point of view, when you are afflicted by tearing thoughts, the miserable feeling you experience, in itself, shows that those tearing thoughts are spiritually 'off'. In the same way, when you fight your tearing thoughts, the peace or the upward shift you attain establishes the validity of fighting them. The validating factor here is not facts, but the considerable improvement in inner feeling.

You should fight your tearing thoughts. When you find your most underlying and pernicious tearing thought, assert the B-Statement powerfully against apparent evidence and against all apparent reason. We have to change the way we speak to ourselves.

Question: The following B-Statements gave me an upward shift: 'I want my dead husband to rise from the dead' and 'I will surely win a billion dollars in the lottery.' Am I kidding myself when I use such statements?

Swamiji: Very clever. You are referring to the upward shift of delusion. That's why we emphasise the A-Statement so much, to base ourselves in practical reality. Even if, as individuals, we have our delusional areas, when we do group-inquiry, the group will provide a rational balancing. Someone in the group is sure to know your husband will not rise from the dead, and you will probably not win a billion dollars in the lottery. They should speak up.

But you know, there's something profound and important in the fact that the dead husband statement gave you an upward shift. I believe that you can find a place where that upward shift intersects with reality, and that will be the place of spiritual power. For example, it may resolve itself as 'I love my husband' or 'I miss my husband' or 'I can contact my husband in the inner world' or 'The Self never dies' or 'My love for him is eternal'. Do you see what I mean? If a highly suspect statement gives a beneficial result (an upward shift), try to deconstruct it in the direction of greater reality.

The same is true when a person has unrealistic goals. The group can help find realistic ones behind the unrealistic ones. It's like touching two wires together. A thing becomes energised when the imagination joins with practical possibility. Some people have lots of imagination and little rational faculty, and others the opposite. The group can fill in the gaps.

B- AND G-STATEMENTS

Question: Could you elaborate on the difference between B- and G-Statements?

Swamiji: A B-Statement is a possibly uplifting statement tailored to your personhood, while the G-Statement is more eternal and impersonal. B-Statements are the set of all possibly uplifting remarks like the famous 'I'm OK-You're OK'. Now the Vedas (Sanskrit texts) don't say that. Well, maybe they do in some way.

G-Statements are statements that express scriptural truths beyond mundane understanding. They might be quotations of scripture, or paraphrasing of the Guru's words or the great yogis'. Gurdjieff calls this 'speaking from the work'.

While you might say that G-Statements are higher on the *matrika* chain than B-Statements, it sometimes happens that a classic G-Statement, like *Tat tvam asi:* 'You are That', is less effective in giving an upward shift than, 'Your essay was very good'. While G-Statements have helped many people on many occasions throughout the ages, even the best of them is not universally effective. I wish it were not this way. Wouldn't it be great if you could say, 'You are That' and everyone became enlightened? Because of the complexity of blocks and obscuring elements, we sometimes have to work more personally by means of B-Statements. A G-Statement can be too far a stretch from where a person is. On the other hand, the search for the G-Statements that have an uplifting effect is particularly worthwhile.

A thumbnail definition is that B-Statements are personally uplifting and situationally uplifting; G-Statements remind the person of their divine nature or divine essence, or the most sublime truth.

A- AND G-STATEMENTS

Question: Is it fair to say that a G-Statement is better than an A-Statement?

Swamiji: Again, I can give you a hearty 'yes' and 'no'. There is a hierarchy of *matrika*; linguistic forms. Some statements point towards the Self and therefore contain more light-truth-energy-love. 'I am Shiva' is a statement with a lot of luminosity while a tearing thought like 'I'm a loser' is a downward shift. In this way, we can see that tearing thoughts and other deluded and ignorant statements are low on the food chain. An A-Statement is much superior to these, and from there we go through B-Statements to G-Statements including mantra, and enter finally into the silence of the Divine. The higher we go, the more energy and the larger our perspective. Just as we see more of the landscape from a higher floor of a building, so a broad mental perspective gives us more energy. Tearing thoughts flow from a contracted point of view. We could call it the 'What about me?' mentality—not much energy in it. G-Statements help you identify with Consciousness or the higher Self and weaken your identification with the personal self.

On the other hand, you don't get right to the top of Mt Everest— you have to pitch base camp. Using the A-Statement as your base camp pulls you out of the maya of tearing thoughts and their nasty friends, and gets you ready to gather your energies for your assault on the summit. So as I've said many times, both have their place.

Question: Could you say something more about the relationship between A- and G-Statements?

Swamiji: A- and G-Statements are fragments of two different narratives about your life, two different ways of thinking about everything that happens to you. Let's look at the issue of death as a clear example. From the point of view of the person, death is the ultimate calamity. It is the most horrible outcome, the thing to be most avoided. It gives rise to A-Statements like 'I am terrified. I will resist this to the end. What will become of me?' and the like. From the point of view of the G-Statement narrative, however, death is not a calamity, but a natural and auspicious event in a larger narrative. I remember reading an *Upanishad* that viewed death from the point of view of the soul, from the top down, rather than from the point of view of the ego, from the bottom up.

The Shiva Process point of view on these two narratives is that both are valid and have their place, even though, one has to say, the impersonal narrative represents a higher truth. The A-Statement is a fragment of the story of the person, the *jiva*, while the G-Statement is a fragment of the Divine; Shiva. Materialists know only the personal narrative and are not aware of Shiva's narrative, thus they're always 'sore beset round' by old age, disease and death. A certain type of spirituality tries to ignore the claims of the person and leaps to the G-Statement. This creates its own problems. The balanced point of view of Shaivite inquiry is to acknowledge both narratives at once. It turns out that by acknowledging the A-Statement narrative, you have a much fuller and easier access to the G-Statement narrative.

THREE SCRIPTS

Question: Are you saying that there are two selves inside each of us?

Swamiji: More than that. As mentioned earlier, Gurdjieff used to say that there are many I's. There's one 'I' when you're happy, one 'I' when you're sad, one 'I' when you're jealous and so on. Each of these I's looks at things differently and makes different decisions. Of course, he said that a master achieves 'permanent I'; that is, a master transcends the ego, which is unstable, and instead connects with the Self. In the Hindu tradition, they call this steady wisdom. In other words, masters remain who they are and are not affected by mood shifts.

Let's think of it a different way. I want to talk about three versions of your life. Let's imagine that three authors have been called in to write your biography. One of them, your worst enemy, writes their script in red ink. It is the story of all your tearing thoughts and worst-case scenarios. It looks at every event in your life through the eye of cynicism and judgment, like Fox News talking about Bill Clinton. The second author is a Zen Buddhist who writes with black ink. He is completely objective and calm. He sees everything as a succession of mental and emotional and physical events: now you say this, now you feel that, now this happens, now that happens. The third writer is a great being who writes in blue ink. He sees everything in your life as part of your process of merging with the Divine. Whatever occurs is part of that process and part of your growth as a spiritual being.

All three scripts have been submitted to the production office in Karma City. Foolishly, they've been mixed up on the same computer program. Our different thought-forms, our different inner voices might be coming from one or the other of these three scripts. The fragments of the red script bring us down and make us miserable. The fragments of the black script are quite grounding and comfortable. The fragments of the blue script are uplifting. Our inquiry discovers and separates these scripts and also distinguishes between the energy and life experience that each one gives.

G-STATEMENTS

Question: I'm not an expert on yogic scriptures so I don't have a fund of G-Statements at hand. Do I need to take a course?

Swamiji: You can find your personal G-Statements by investigating your own life. Here's what you can try. Remember the best time of your life; maybe it was a period in high school, maybe it was a summer vacation, maybe it was the first two months of a new relationship. In meditation, think about that time, get in touch with the feeling that you had and then see what thoughts you were speaking to yourself then. Those thoughts will act as self-generated G-Statements. All right, maybe technically they're B-Statements, but they come from the scripture of your own soul. As we can use false A-Statements as B-Statements in regard to our chief fault, so too can we use B-Statements as G-Statements. The point is, they once put you in, or accompanied, a pristine state of consciousness, which, if you could attain permanently, would make you a great being. If you can contact the self-talk you had then, you will learn a lot about yourself. Find that self-talk, adapt it to your present situation and work with it. What was the 'background music' you were playing during the time of greatest happiness?

Question: I have a problem with G-Statements. Maybe it reflects my problem with authority, but I keep wanting to ask, 'Who says I am Shiva?'

Swamiji: Some time after the Renaissance, Western culture moved from a religious world view to a scientific one. Deductive reasoning (from the top down), which had held sway for centuries, was severely questioned and replaced by inductive reasoning (from the bottom up). Science is inductive in that it works with concrete particulars and does not trust general statements without first proving them. Religions don't usually need proof; they give big statements and say, 'God said this'. They call it scripture—whichever one they espouse. But science has been so victorious that we in the West are automatically suspicious of any authority at all. Yogis will say that these G-Statements actually come from higher Consciousness. They were revealed to sages in deep states of meditation. I think this is true, but you might still have a problem with that.

Why don't you look at it this way? G-Statements can be used inductively, in that you can consider them to be experiments. G-Statements are valid, not because Shankaracharya or Ramana said them, but only when they create a sense of harmony, peace or upliftment when dropped into your inner world. See, now you're an inner scientist and have a criterion by which you can test these statements objectively.

One of the problems with large top-down statements like 'I am Shiva' is that they don't work for everyone. If they worked for everyone, they would be a panacea and we wouldn't need God. Because of our individual differences, different keys unlock our doors. An important part of our yoga is to find which precise key works for each of us. You may hear the teaching, 'I am Shiva', and it doesn't quite feel right and you could spend years beating yourself up because you don't resonate with 'I am Shiva'; that would be absurd.

On the other hand, maybe the G-Statement 'God loves me' gives you instant peace. By all means, go with it. Respect your individual differences and don't attack yourself. The secret is not to try to make *every* type of yoga work for you but to find *one* yoga that does work for you. In this sense, we each have to find our inner guru. My Guru told me to contemplate 'I am Shiva' and because it struck a chord in me, it worked perfectly. Despite how great he was, if he had told me something that was not meaningful to my inner nature, it would not have stuck with me for so many years. In this way, we are ultimately our own guru because inevitably we make our own selection from among the instructions that the outer Guru gives us.

Both the inductive and deductive approaches are necessary for our full development. There is no intrinsic reason why they have to be at war. Deductive statements are statements of faith and they affirm higher Consciousness. Inductive statements are statements of intelligence and discernment and they acknowledge what is so. G-Statements are deductive and A-Statements are inductive.

I HAVE GREAT IDEAS BUT I CAN'T THINK OF THEM

Question: Just today in our inquiry group, a feeling was nagging at me. But despite our best efforts with many kinds of statements, we couldn't get to the bottom of it. Is it possible that sometimes a thing needs to 'cook' and you can only discover what it is about later?

Swamiji: That is very true. The Spanish explorer Balboa could not see the Pacific until he got to the last hill. No amount of craning his neck would do the job. Of course, he must have smelled the salt air and seen the seagulls, so he knew he was getting close to a body of water. Knowledge is a lot like that. It comes in bits. We are talking here of revelation, and revelation is that which is revealed by Consciousness. In doing inquiry, the point is to come as close as you can to what is so and what is real in your experience with your present wisdom and technology. This leads to some charming and zany statements like 'This is a work in progress' or 'I understand as much of it as I can at the moment' or 'This feeling is not ripe' or the classic Shiva Process statement, 'There is something I need to say, but I don't know what it is'. Isn't that a wonderful statement?

If you are astute, you can use this idea to bring contentment in all kinds of betwixt and between situations. Consider, for example, similar statements like 'There is a step I have to take spiritually, but I don't know what it is' or 'I am willing to take the next step, but I don't know what it is' or 'There is a good way of regarding this situation, but I don't know what it is' or 'I invoke a new way of looking at this situation'. Do you get the drift of this sort of technique? Like Tukaram, you make everything work for you. I should give my father a footnote here, because I suspect this bit of lateral thinking is based on my father's oft-repeated remark, 'I have great ideas but I can't think of them'.

For Balboa, the right statement would have been, 'I think I'm close to the sea, but I can't see it yet'. And then at the crest of the last hill, he could have said, 'I see the sea'. Each would have been an A-Statement that would have accurately described his present experience.

Why is this worth doing? This is the study of your own awareness. *Chaitanyamatma*: 'You are your awareness.' You can know about the moon and Mars and science and religion and history and philosophy and government and chemistry and food. But if you don't know about yourself, then there is a big hole in your knowledge. So when we study awareness, we are studying who we really are. To know how awareness expands and contracts is very important; why there is more illumination, less illumination; more happiness, less happiness. All these things are important. And this is a method of looking directly at it. It can be looked at *directly* and that is what we do in good Self-inquiry. We look directly into the face of Consciousness.

CARROT IN MY EAR

Question: Would you talk a little more about the unconscious?

Swamiji: Yes, let me discuss the unconscious with reference to my metaphor, having a 'carrot in your ear'. A carrot in your ear is from a story I heard in high school. Two fellows are walking along the street and one says to the other, 'You have a carrot in your ear!' and the other says, 'I can't hear you, I have a carrot in my ear'. This joke has reverberated for me down the years. It is central to group-inquiry. To have a carrot in your ear means there is something that you are not hearing. It is a technical term here. Each of us has a carrot in our ear about something. We hide some things from ourselves; that is, we put them into the unconscious.

Our previous conditioning shows up in dysfunctional, repetitive behaviour. It is always fraught with negative emotion such as fear or disgust. It is not rational and causes us harm. The intense focus of the Self-inquiry group brings Consciousness to bear on these hidden patterns and helps participants expand their awareness until they can see what they are doing. In the crucible of conscious focus, what was previously hidden becomes revealed. It is these hidden patterns that create repetitive behaviour. We go round and round in the same circle.

The first step is to remove carrots from our ears. This expands our mind and creates new understandings. Messages are always coming to us from inside and outside. They are there in what other people say and indicate to us, and also in the form of impulses from within. When the carrot is gone, we begin to hear and pay attention to those messages. Interestingly, the first step in the classical path of *jnana* is *hearing* the truth. But it is not enough just to be a thinker; you should feel too. It is also not enough to be a thinker and a feeler; you should be a doer too. What you think and feel should translate into action. When the group recommends an action, a D-Statement, it should be followed up. Homework is an essential part of the process.

There was one woman whose play led the group through the misery and difficulties of her life. After grappling with the murkiness of it all, the group would always come up with the same thing: 'Get a job!' Each time the group got there, it was like making a new discovery. And then they would realise that the same discovery was made last week, and the week before also. The homework was always the same, but she never did get a job. It became impossible for her to continue in group work because she wasn't taking the step that she needed to take. She was wasting the group's energy and goodwill by leading it down the same primrose path each session. I am suggesting that there are a number of ways to make the unconscious conscious. One is by using the feedback of the group as revelation, and another is to follow the group's suggestion to take action in an area of insecurity or confusion.

FACING THE TRUTH

Question: I was feeling good until something happened in the group that affected me. I don't even know if I would call it a downward shift, but I was very stirred up. I saw that it brought a lot of things up that were important for me to understand. I see that what looks bad in the short run might really be valuable in the long run.

Swamiji: Very good, that is the right attitude. You are echoing an old yogic aphorism that says pleasure-seeking is sweet in the beginning and bitter in the end, while yogic discipline is bitter in the beginning but sweet in the end. When I lived in Ganeshpuri with my teacher for about three years, it was not a bed of roses. I faced so many things and it was such a crucifixion—and he didn't give a damn! In fact, he liked it! You gain a lot of rewards by facing the spiritual truth.

SUMMARY

- Group-inquiry is like a ritual that follows a certain procedure to expand Consciousness.

- Group-inquiry differs from *satsang* because it seeks blocks in order to undo them.

- Divine Shiva Process works directly with awareness.

- Feedback can reveal our unconscious.

- Group process uses multiple points of view.

- Life itself is a larger group process; a feedback system.

- Group-inquiry creates a discipline on speech.

- The goal of group-inquiry is to unblock awareness, not to fix people.

- A zinger is feedback with an unexpectedly powerful effect.

- Group-inquiry does not encourage unsolicited advice.

- The D-Statement is a doing statement or homework.

- In the group process, the player receives A-, B-, G- and D-Statements.

- While therapy focuses on the person, group-inquiry focuses on the upward shift of Consciousness.

- The inquiry group builds a mandala of feeling.

- In group-inquiry, we observe the contractions and expansions of Consciousness caused by *matrika*.

- Shifting statements indicate a connection between the human and the Divine.

- In group-inquiry, listen with your true Self rather than your mind.

- To give feedback, access your feeling and offer it as though it were the player's feeling.

- The group should pace its feedback.

- Feedback is an offering not a telling.

- The Shiva Process upward shift is comparable to the chod sacrifice.

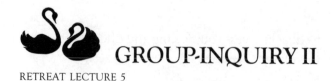 GROUP-INQUIRY II

Rama, such is this forest known as world-appearance; he who cuts its very root with the axe of inquiry is freed from it. Some arrive at this understanding soon, others after a very long time.

Yoga Vashishta

The state of liberation is not confined to any special heavenly abode, nor does it imply an ascension towards such a heavenly abode. Liberation is the illumining of one's divine power attainable by means of untying the knots of ignorance.

Abhinavagupta

THE SCHOLAR OF Kashmir Shaivism, Mark Dyczkowski, elegantly summarises the process of spiritual growth that is the point of both personal inquiry and group-inquiry. He says:

> The yogi [of Kashmir Shaivism] treads the path of Consciousness expansion. The movement from the contracted to the expanded state marks the transition from ignorance to understanding, from [contraction] ... to a direct, intuitive awareness of the unity and integral wholeness of our own [true] nature.

This movement of expansion from contraction highlights the spiritual kinship between Shiva Process and Kashmir Shaivism. Without reference to Shaivism, a number of metaphors can help us gain an overview of Shiva Process.

THE VISION QUEST

The Shiva Process group is a journey through varied terrain. It passes through verdant fields and through wastelands and deserts. It winds into the mountains and down into the valleys. Sometimes, it feels as though direction has been lost and there is no map available. Like the archetypal journey of the hero, its goal is the holy grail of bliss-consciousness. The landscape is defined by the feeling content and energy level of the group in any moment. While the goal may be far off, the voyagers orient themselves by the A-Statement, using it as the ancient travellers used the stars.

THE ELECTRICAL CIRCUIT

A second metaphor is that of the electrical circuit. Think of energy flowing around a circuit into which appliances are connected. Each appliance has 'resistance', an electrical term that sounds like Shiva Process jargon. Resistance blocks the energy; it diminishes the energy in the whole circuit.

Resistance in an electrical circuit is analogous to second force or the blocks that people carry in the group. There is an energy that circulates through the group and when participants have blocks, that energy is blocked. A person's blocks keep them from being fully present to the group enterprise. Their attention is undermined by the block. Their mind is off somewhere, involved consciously or unconsciously in some other situation or state of suffering. The task of the group is to unblock the energy and uplift it.

Each participant, like an appliance, manifests a certain amount of resistance. As the group work goes on, resistance is overcome and the flow of energy increases. Resistance is created by wrong understanding which manifests in speech. When the spoken word is in harmony with Self, then flow is well established. Ramana, using the same metaphor, regards silence as the perfect culmination of speech. It is not the silence of blocked expression, but the silence of wordless communion.

Ramana says:

> Silence is ever-speaking; it is a perennial flow of language; it is interrupted by speaking. These words obstruct that

mute language. There is electricity flowing in a wire. With resistance to its passage, it glows as a lamp or revolves as a fan. In the wire it remains as electric energy. Similarly also, silence is the eternal flow of language, obstructed by words.

What one fails to know by conversation extending to several years can be known in a trice in Silence [Consciousness].

That is the highest and most effective language.

THE MIRROR

A third metaphor is that of the mirror: in the group, everyone mirrors everyone. The space in the centre of the group is a shining mirror of Consciousness. Maybe that is why we crave relationship, because when we see another in front of us, it intensifies awareness. Consciousness is looking at Consciousness. When conscious beings put their attention on each other with love, Consciousness intensifies. In the group, Consciousness is intensified and in that intensification, energy is increased. Consciousness is raised to new understandings. It ups the game—'supercharges' it. This mirroring also serves to reflect the unconscious back to us. That is what happens in a relationship or marriage: you get your unconscious fed back to you by your partner, sometimes in a harsh way. It is perhaps the essence of spirituality to uncover what we hold in our unconscious. It is great work.

THE DETECTIVE STORY

A fourth metaphor is that of a detective story. The detective story presents a simple universe in which you go through darkness into light, and you don't get bogged down by personal issues. It is about bad guys getting caught: you discover clues and you get to the truth. To a yogi, life is a detective story and there is always a deeper truth to be discovered. A related metaphor is that of peeling an onion, stripping away the outer layers and getting to the essence.

Shiva Process is a path of energy. To follow the energy, you have to let go of attachments and prejudices which take you on false trails with diminished energy. It's a little like Hansel and Gretel following the breadcrumbs through the woods.

LAYABHAVANA

In *Consciousness Is Everything*, I talk about a process called *layabhavana*, which is described in the *Shiva Sutras*:

> *Sharire samharaha kalanam*

> The forces or *tattvas* in the body should be dissolved backwards into the Source.

Kashmir Shaivism describes creation as an emanation from pure Consciousness. The one Consciousness steps down through 36 levels, ultimately becoming the material world. Even though the 36th *tattva* or level is the most gross, it also has within it all the other 35 levels. Thus, Consciousness exists even at the core of a stone, though particularly well hidden. *Layabhavana* progresses inward and therefore up the evolutionary scale, moving from the material outer layer to the conscious core.

In Shiva Process, we follow this model, resolving the gross into the subtle, always seeking more energy and more light. Blocks appear because we are stuck. As we inquire, we irradiate the dense area of the block with the light that is actually underneath. This movement or resolution of the gross into the subtle, of the less conscious into the more conscious, is *layabhavana*.

Patanjali gives a similar teaching in the *Yoga Sutras*. In order to overcome the afflictions of life, the yogi resolves them backwards to their source.

> *Te pratiprasava-heyaha sukshmaha*

> These, the subtle ones, can be reduced by resolving them backward into their origin.

If we think of evolution as a progressive movement from simple to complex, inert to more conscious, the principle of Self-inquiry goes in the opposite direction. Here, the deeper we go by 'backward reference' towards the subject, the more spacious and conscious the terrain.

THE YAGNA

An aspirant, enlightened by such realization, should offer all his conceptual functions and ideas to the sacrificial fire of pure consciousness of the self, kindled highly by the winds of the self-contemplative yoga, becoming one with such fire.

Abhinavagupta

Finally, there is for me the principal metaphor: the *yagna;* a Vedic ritual. In this ritual, which lies at the heart of the Hindu religion, Brahmin priests sit around a sacred fire and throw ghee (clarified butter) and other foodstuffs into it, while reciting mantras. When the ghee hits the fire, it flares up. The participants in group-inquiry are like modern-day Brahmins, sitting around the fire of Consciousness. The group begins in separation, and by making A-Statements the circle is joined—when you make an A-Statement you come into relationship with the process, the ritual. As you make B-Statements, you throw ghee on the flame and Consciousness is raised.

From this point of view, group-inquiry is a sacrament. This does not mean it should be undertaken in the ponderous manner of many 'religious' ceremonies, but rather in the serious yet light-hearted style of Hindu ritual. I have written a few aphorisms relating group-inquiry to the Vedic fire ritual:

The centre is the fire.

The centre is Consciousness.

The centre, here, refers to the space enclosed by the people in the circle of inquiry. All dialogue takes place in that space, and words and conversations enter and cross that space, from mouth to ear. These aphorisms apply also to life as a whole—in any relationship, the space between two people is that centre. The space between two people in a relationship is critical for the relationship. Is that space full of strife and separation? Or is that space vibrating with love and upliftment? Many a relationship begins in expansion and love and then becomes contracted. What a mystery!

My Self-realised chow-chow, Bhakti, used to always plant herself in the very centre of every Shiva Process group, which she made sure not to miss. She was sensitive to the Shakti and loved that conscious centre.

Words of truth brighten the fire.

Words of love brighten the fire.

What goes into that space? Words and feelings go into that space, and they are precisely what contract or expand that space. Words of truth and love quicken and vivify the experience.

The player is the priest.

I offer myself to the fire of Consciousness.

I honour each one as they are; may they offer themselves to Consciousness.

This is the *yagna* metaphor. The inner purpose of the *yagna* of inquiry is to uplift and make the fire blaze brighter; that is, to make the fire of awareness blaze brighter. Truth and love are the two ingredients that make the fire blaze brighter. As the work goes on, it becomes clear whether the fire is blazing bright or not.

It's not surprising that the *yagna* is a good metaphor for the Shiva Process. It also reminds us of the previously mentioned *chod* practice, in which the body of the practitioner is metaphorically offered as sacrificial food to hungry deities, thus achieving an upward shift. Similarly, the private space of the Shiva Process practitioner's ego is sacrificed into the fire of the group process.

SHIVA PROCESS OPENING STATEMENTS

Gurdjieff used to say, 'Remember why you came'. He had that sign up in his ashram. When people first come to an ashram, they are on fire for wisdom, for the truth, for God and Self-knowledge. Then they get caught up in the routine of the ashram and the pettiness of personalities and lose some of that original fire. You would do well to reaffirm your spiritual purpose every day—to say to yourself, 'I want to know the Self. I want to get close to the Shakti. I want to know God. Today I will live in accord with the highest truth'. That is why Gurdjieff said, 'Remember why you came'. That initial reason is the underlying cause, the pure intentionality of your quest, and it is always operating, even when you seem to lose sight of it.

Also, when we do group-inquiry, it is good to reaffirm our purpose at the beginning of every session. We do this by means of the following opening statements. They are like opening mantras at the beginning of a ritual. The group leader reads them out and the participants silently connect with each statement.

I dedicate myself to speaking the truth.

This statement implies participation. It is necessary to participate. You have to give your value. When we play it safe and hold back and don't speak up, we are not really living. A recurring theme in Henry James' novels is the degree to which people are dead-in-life. The goal of his central characters is to live life more fully. If we don't contribute, we become alienated: we complain behind the scenes and get angry at others and ourself. You have to live like a riverboat gambler—you have to take a risk. Don't play it close to the vest; speak up, give your value! Our worst fear is to look stupid, so an effective exercise is to *try* to look stupid. I have given that assignment several times. It is extremely freeing. One ancient branch of Shaivism practised exactly that as a spiritual method. You don't have to go that far, but you must participate.

When we dedicate ourselves to speaking the truth, we are also dedicating ourselves to speaking up. You dishonour your Shiva nature if you don't think that your perception, your understanding, is valuable and valid. Because some participants speak up too much and some too little, I've been experimenting with a method of giving feedback that balances these tendencies. In this method, at the time of giving A-Statement feedback, the leader asks the group to go inside and come up with an A-Statement for the player. Then, each member gives their feedback, even when it repeats earlier feedback. This disciplines the overly enthusiastic and includes and reaches out to the shy. So far, results are promising. This is an alternative method of giving feedback, which may indeed become our standard practice. The same method can be used in giving B-Statements. Every person, as Shiva, has their own angle on reality, and has a valuable contribution to the whole. It is like a musical piece: if one instrument is not playing, there is a lack.

I dedicate myself to speaking the truth with kindness.

I have already discussed the polarity of truth and kindness. In Sanskrit, they are *satya* (truth) and *ahimsa* (kindness). They are two of the *yamas*; yogic restraints. Gandhi, of course, is associated with *ahimsa*, which is non-violence, here translated as kindness. Non-violence by itself can be weak and flabby; truth by itself can be harsh and cruel. They must marry. Truth and kindness must be present in equal measure.

I dedicate myself to helping others know the true Self.

Another way of saying this is 'I offer myself to serve others' which hints at the element of sacrifice and self-offering in group work. Some people think that if they don't have a problem, they shouldn't be in an inquiry group. This is wrong understanding. As I've mentioned, if you are in a great inner state: serve, help. That is the highest path. Those who serve others will have all their needs met. Everything will come to them; they won't have to worry about themselves. We spend so much time worrying about ourselves: 'Are we getting our share? Is someone else getting more?' It is much better to serve—to serve others and serve the process.

I dedicate myself to knowing the true Self.

I rededicate myself to the essence of sadhana.

I honour everything that arises as the play of Consciousness.

No mind movements are excluded from Consciousness. Everything is there in Consciousness—the whole of creation. Every bit of it has been spun out of divinity; every bit of this creation, not only the good stuff. So, 'I honour everything' does not mean I have to accept everything or that I cannot choose or I don't know good from bad—it does not mean that at all. My ability to know good from bad and my desire for good rather than bad also arises from Consciousness and should be honoured as well.

Shaivism teaches that the Self or Consciousness is the core of every person, thing and event. It stands to reason, then, that everything that arises is a new opportunity to connect with its core reality; the Self. When things go against our preference or plan, it becomes difficult to find that blissful core. But remembering, in principle, that the essence is always discoverable, the yogi of inquiry, a devotee of the play of Consciousness, enjoys the challenge.

A yogi has a different ethical perspective from a moralist. For a yogi, good and bad do not refer to a particular moral code. Good is that which brings one closer to God or the Self, and bad is that which takes one away. To know which is which is classical yogic discrimination; *viveka*. To let go of what is bad is yogic dispassion; *vairagya*. And to adhere to what is good is devotion; *bhakti*.

I carefully watch the movement of Shakti within and without.

Now we come to the heart of the matter. In group-inquiry, as in personal inquiry, we watch the subtle play of energy in every moment, in every word. We watch the energy expand and contract. We watch our reactions.

And finally,

I seek the highest wisdom in each situation.

There are many levels, many lenses through which to view things. Our perspective can be personal or cosmic. While not excluding personal and specific understandings, we also commit ourselves to the highest perspective in every situation. We don't have to remind ourselves to view things personally—that happens automatically—but we do well to commit and recommit ourselves to a higher point of view.

These, then, are the opening statements. In every human action, there is the physical or outer-world activity and also the inner-world intention, which is all-important. The knife cuts a person. Is it the surgeon's knife that wishes to heal, or the murderer's knife that wishes to kill? Our intentionality shapes the meaning of our life.

Sometimes we hide our intention from ourselves. We might think we are being kind to someone, but underneath we are really 'having a go' at them. We keep this subtle fact hidden from ourselves, but it is discoverable through inquiry. It is good to know and acknowledge what you are really doing. If you are going to have a go at someone, it is important that you know you are having a go. Then you can decide whether the consequences are worth it or not. It is useful to rededicate ourselves through these beginning statements. It sharpens the instrument. We become more 'on purpose'.

ADDITIONAL OPENING STATEMENTS

In cases in which a Shiva Process group has many inexperienced participants or the leader feels a lack of authority, an additional set of opening statements can be used to indicate guidelines and give support to the leader, as outlined below.

By group consensus we agree to:

- Respect the Shiva Process discipline.

- Make A- and B-Statements as offered.

- Offer all feedback in the spirit of investigation and experimentation.

- Offer all feedback free of judgment and personal agenda.

- Give advice only when solicited.

- Be guided by the appointed leader.

The group leader can select from among these if they seem valuable, and give them before or after the normal opening statements.

SHIVA PROCESS CLOSING QUESTIONS

Hindu rituals begin with an invocation, using certain mantras. The end of a ritual is marked by another set of mantras. In this way, the ritual is set apart as a sacred space in time. In the same way, group-inquiry is sacralised. While it's true that all of life is inquiry in which the same laws apply, it also serves a good purpose to think of the inquiry group as a special, sacred time. There we bring a higher and purer intention and an increased attentiveness.

To 'seal the group off', I use the Vedic mantra:

Om *Purnamadah purnamidam*
Purnat purnamudachyate
Purnasya purnamadaya
Purnameva vashishyate
Om *shantih, shantih, shantih.*

That is perfect, this is perfect.
From the perfect, the perfect comes.
If you take the perfect from the perfect, the perfect
remains.
Om, peace, peace, peace.

Everyone chants these mantras together. It suggests that whatever has happened in the group has been a play of Consciousness. It calls attention to the underlying and ever-available perfection at every stage of the Shiva Process. After the mantras formally end the group, the closing statements are made.

If the opening statements look forward to the task at hand and hone our attention, the closing questions look back at what has taken place and examine the results. Sometimes you carry away negative feeling from the group. Or there may be a sense of something unfinished—a lack of resolution. An element of risk exists in doing this work. But while we may not always be uplifted, we can always learn something.

To maximise resolution, I have designed a series of questions for the leader to read out at the end of each group. The leader reads them one at a time and group members raise their hands without comment if the statement applies to them. A lot of information emerges. The group is now over. These questions are a kind of closing ritual.

The first question is:

Are you carrying anything?

We immediately address the possibility that something may have been picked up in the hurly-burly of the group.

Did you see more than you said?

People don't speak up for a variety of reasons, which we have started to address in the group through alternative means of giving feedback, as mentioned earlier. Some can't find the words, some are afraid of expressing themselves. These self-disenfranchised ones are given another opportunity to speak up by raising their hands to this question. Having seen the hands, a leader, seeking to increase the 'truth' quotient of the group, might ask, 'What did you see that you didn't say?' I often refrain from this possibility because of the risk of a downward shift, but it is an option that can be taken.

Do you want to praise anyone?

Do you want to blame anyone?

This is the awards ceremony. Here the focus is on the amount of truth that people brought to the process. Again, the leader might ask a participant to name someone they want to praise or blame. Blaming here does not mean irresponsible dumping of anger; rather, it is a means of pointing out a mistake that may have been made, such as withholding feedback, withdrawing or, alternatively, dominating the process, or offloading negative feelings onto another.

Are you worried about anyone?

The leader asks, 'Who are you worried about?' A group member answers, 'I am worried about X, Y and Z'. And that is sufficient.

Did you want to say anything to anyone?

Were you able to say what you needed to say?

These questions are designed to empower those who can't or won't speak up. Once again, the leader might choose those who raise their hands to speak.

Was there truth?

Was there falsity?

I have never seen the hands up for falsity outnumber the hands up for truth, but that doesn't mean that it couldn't happen. There are times when the group wanders lost in confusion and can't find its way out. Ending the group is then like sleep at the end of a bad day. The slate is wiped clean and we can start over next time.

Do you want to apologise to anyone?

Here's an opportunity to equalise any karmas that have arisen.

Did anger, fear or sadness arise in you or in the group?

This question simply calls attention to the ebb and flow of emotions that has inevitably taken place.

Did the group touch a mystery?

A lot of what happens in a group transcends the mind. And this leads us to a higher octave of the same question, my favourite question:

Did you see God or evidence of God?

A lovely question that invites the participants to interpret it in any way they like.

Was there equal measure of truth and kindness?

When truth outweighs kindness, the group is interesting but dangerous. When kindness outweighs truth, the group tends to be safe but boring.

Were you present: All? A lot? Some? Little?

Did the feeling move up? Did the feeling move down?

These questions invite the participants to examine their own experience and increase their awareness of the movement of the group.

What was the high point of the group in feeling and interest?

When did the group peak? When was the most superb moment? I might ask a specific person what their high point was.

Do you have advice for anyone?

As we've said, the Shiva Process is not about giving unsolicited advice, but, instead, about helping people discover the right path (their own advice within themselves).

Did you have a yogic or practical understanding?

Do you or does anyone need homework?

D-Statements, homework, are a necessary part of the process. Homework implies taking understandings and putting them into action. It is only when understandings are acted on, *lived*, that they become metaphysically real. When a new perspective or a new understanding is gained, a bit of challenging homework is much to the point. Or else you encounter the disheartening phenomenon of a person having the same realisation over and over but never moving forward.

These questions clean up and tie up the group. A leader can explore any of them, but simply asking for a show of hands in answer to each question is a magical way to resolve things.

Self-inquiry has wide application. It can be used anywhere for anything. It can be used in all four areas of life—to address a physical problem, a block in your career or relationship, or a spiritual problem.

The head of the women's golf team at a distinguished Melbourne Golf Club came to *satsang* here. She asked me and some others to come to the club to work with the team. I felt like a sports psychologist. You can imagine that a few of my universes came together there. Among other things, I asked them to imagine themselves standing on the tee of a hole that was uncomfortable for them. I said, 'Close your eyes, you are on the third tee. Where is the feeling? Is there tension in the navel?' It was very interesting. I asked them to make statements and they had shifts. Afterwards, I heard they had made golf progress.

Whatever the issue is, in whatever part of your life, you can focus on that issue and connect with it in your feeling. Feelings and thoughts will arise and you can work with them. A lot of information will come to you.

PROXYING

We have finished the main outline of how group-inquiry flows. Now I will talk about the important related technique called *proxying*. I discovered it after a phone call from a man, let me call him Chip. Certain people are unpleasant to speak with because of unprocessed or unconscious emotions they carry and transmit—Chip was one of those.

As I spoke with him on that occasion, I began to feel the familiar unpleasant sensations. On the surface, everything was polite and correct, but underneath, something else was going on. He was wearing a mask. When I hung up, I felt contaminated by his unspoken feeling. My first impulse was to throw it back at him angrily, but I had a flash of insight that revealed another possibility.

I reasoned: I was feeling fine when I began to speak with him, then I felt contaminated. Somehow Chip had come into me. I didn't know whether I had allowed him in by feeling sympathy for him, or by means of having a negative reaction to him. Either way, I was 'carrying' him. I sat down and said, 'I am Chip'; I identified with him. Assuming that the feeling I was carrying was from him, I made statements within myself as though I were him. I let his feeling express itself as A-Statements, and they surprised me. It was like experiencing Chip from within himself. All his tearing thoughts came up: 'I am unlovable. I am lonely. I am unworthy.' I said them all within myself as they arose. Then I made B-Statements like 'Please love me. I am worthy'. In this way, I accepted Chip and his energy. When I didn't push him away from me, the feeling moved up through me. It went up and out through my *sahasrara*, and I felt completely clear and free of it. That was the discovery of proxying. Later, Chip said he felt better after our phone call. In fact, it felt better for me, too, to accept and process Chip within myself rather than reject him.

Proxying is a mysterious technique that reflects the essential oneness of the Self. While another's inner space is private and theirs alone, it can be approached through empathy. It is an act of love and sacrifice. Unconsciously, Chip exuded a negative feeling from which people fled. He felt constantly rejected and that rejection increased his tearing thoughts about being unlovable.

It was a vicious cycle of despair. My first thought, too, had been to angrily reject him and throw off the negative feeling I was picking up. Instead, by proxying him, I accepted his feeling—and therefore him—and moved it through me. I can't brag too much about this, since Jesus did the same thing for the whole world, and Lord Shiva did it by drinking the poison of the universe.

In proxying, you stand in for a person who is not able to move their own feeling. Or you may proxy a person who is difficult for you. Then you see the situation from within that person. It looks different from that person's perspective than it looks from yours. I have talked previously about giving bad feedback, where you say, for example, 'I am X and I am full of ego'. Of course, X is not saying, 'I am full of ego' within. Here, your 'feedback' is actually your judgment of X. To find out what is actually going on in their inner world, you would have to tune in to it or ask them. So, a person like Chip might make you want to say, 'You are disgusting', but inside he is saying, 'I am unlovable. I am unworthy' to himself.

Proxying is a compassionate act. You merge with that person and look from within them, as it were, with sympathy. Nobody looks like a monster from within. Another person can judge them, but deep within they feel worthy of love. Maybe their mother loved them, and they have justifications for all their bad actions.

Not only is proxying compassionate, it is also practical. Because of attachment, vulnerability, openness or aversion, you sometimes get affected by the feelings of another person. Whatever the reason, you come away from an encounter filled with bad feeling. Next time this happens, try this experiment: sit down, assume the feeling is the other person's, then proxy it, making statements for the other person. If such a treatment creates movement, you would be justified in saying that it had indeed belonged to the other person.

Here in the ashram, there is a strong culture of Shiva Process. That is good, of course, but, as with any culture, it can have a downside. It emerges when students blame their negative feeling on others as in, 'You dumped your anger on me', which is then met with 'No, you dumped your anger on me first'. This is a vice of Shiva Process. It should be understood that once a feeling is in you, it's yours. You wouldn't get another person's feeling if you weren't in some way vulnerable to them. Being aware of this pitfall, you can treat certain feelings as another person's and proxy them. As a safeguard, you should experiment with finding A- and B-Statements, as if the feeling is your own. If you get no shift, you can then try proxying.

If you want to use the technique of proxying, there is one distinction to make. Proxying works best when you actually get in touch with feeling and make statements relevant to that feeling. It's not the same as giving a person a psychic reading in which you *mentally* project into the person's feeling. It's hard to convey this distinction, but it is an important one. The wrong path is when you give what you *think* they are feeling, rather than making statements from *your actual feeling*, which you can assume *relates to theirs*.

You can proxy anyone—public figures like presidents or filmmakers—and make real discoveries of the structure of *matrika* they hold. You can even proxy nations and institutions. We once proxied the National Gallery of Victoria, and it was as though it spoke to us. The language and the feeling are all there hanging in the ether. You could proxy, for example, the White House, the Kremlin or Graceland, in the same way.

TRACK 11. INQUIRY:
THE MARVELLOUS TECHNIQUE OF PROXYING

You can proxy another person when that person's feeling invades you or when you are a well-wisher of that person and you want to help them. In either of these cases, proxying has a magical effect.

Since Consciousness is one, we can work with another's feeling inside of ourselves and we can help another in this way and we also can decontaminate ourselves when we've been affected by another's feeling. Use proxying.

To proxy, you look at the feeling within you and you assume that it comes from the other person and you make statements, as you would for yourself. You begin with A-Statements. You say, 'I'm X ...'—X being the other person—'and I feel angry. I feel sad. I feel scared'. You can be specific and find their underlying statements. 'I'm X, I feel unlovable. I'm X, I feel weak. I'm X, I feel like a failure.' To help the other person, when you come to the end of the A-Statements, you can make B-Statements. 'I'm X and I feel optimistic. I'm X, I am capable. I'm X, I love myself.' You can go seamlessly into G-Statements. 'I'm X and I am Shiva.'

INTERNAL AND EXTERNAL CONSIDERING

External considering (positive reflection): to give love and understanding unconditionally to another without attachment or aversion. To reflect their true Self to them. 'Taking things impersonally.'

Internal considering (negative reflection): to internalise a false version of another person or a false 'I' because of attachment or aversion. To reflect a distorted version of another within yourself. 'Taking things personally.'

Gurdjieff's brilliant ideas, internal and *external considering*, are useful in terms of proxying. External considering involves speaking to people where they're at, taking into consideration their attitudes, opinions and values, as well as their emotional situation. It is a form of respect and even worship. Proxying is related to external considering.

I learned my best lessons in external considering by watching my Guru's interactions with an endless stream of people on a daily basis. It was fascinating for me to observe him because, to my eyes, he met each one exactly where they were.

To truly externally consider, you have to 'get off' your own stuff and be available to the other. This makes you free. It is uplifting both for you and the other person, hence, Gurdjieff enjoins us to always practise external considering.

When impressions come into awareness, if there is not attachment or aversion, they pass through and don't stick. Attachment and aversion are emotional terms, two kinds of negative emotions, and they are the glue that creates internal considering or negative reflection. Detachment leads to positive reflection or external considering where the reflection of the other person is not allowed to enter into you, but reflects benignly back to them.

That Gurdjieff put a sign up, 'Externally consider always, internally consider never' gives you some idea. Internal considering has many forms, among them worrying about what other people think of you or feeling that people don't give you enough credit or, in fact, don't consider you enough. The common feature behind all the forms of internal considering is that your inner space becomes contaminated when you internally considering another person. Here, instead of simply reflecting the other person back to them, you take things personally and allow them to enter you in a way that is ultimately harmful.

Your inner world belongs to you alone. No one should be in that space besides the Self, or if you practise devotional yoga, the deity, the beloved, who is actually not different from your Self. I've already said that no one can enter your inner space but you, so when I say someone comes into your space, I don't mean they actually enter that space, but that you have become disempowered by wrongly considering another, and your space has become tainted. A follower of the path of Samkhya would say the conscious Self has become contaminated by matter. Internal considering allows matter (other people) in.

I remember a story a contemporary poet told of hearing Robert Frost give a poetry class at his university. As background, you have to know that Frost and T.S. Eliot were deadly rivals. In his class, Frost asked his students to read some of their poetry and then he critiqued them. One woman read a poem and Frost asked her with considerable emotion, 'Who wrote that poem?' She said, 'I did'. He said, 'No, who *really* wrote that poem?' She was nonplussed. Finally, he said with scorn, 'T.S. Eliot'. He was saying that T.S. Eliot had unwittingly entered her poetry space. Presumably, Eliot had entered her space because she admired him. Others might enter our inner space not through admiration, but for negative reasons.

Many things weaken you so that you wrongly let in another. Every one of the negative emotions can create its own kind of internal considering. Whenever you're angry at another person, or fearful or jealous, you let that person in. Your tearing thoughts might be the presence of your parents or some long-dead ancestor making themselves felt in your inner space. In the Robert Frost story, it is possible that the woman had tearing thoughts about her own poetic talents, and felt, unconsciously, that only by echoing Eliot would she be worthy. Internal considering is never beneficial.

The various desires and fears that intrude on our inner space are like false voices; false I's that have penetrated our inner world. Our task is to disregard these false voices and know the voice of the Self. Because of our reactions to events and people in our lives, negative and positive impressions enter us and speak within us. It becomes appropriate, then, to ask the odd-sounding question, 'Who has entered my inner space?'

TRACK 12.
INQUIRY: WHO HAS ENTERED MY INNER SPACE?

The next time you feel depressed, unbalanced or contracted, turn your attention inside, become aware of the state of your inner world, and ask yourself, 'Who is in here?' or 'Who have I let in?' You will be surprised at what you understand from this simple inquiry.

Hint: If there's someone with whom you're somewhat obsessed, or even thinking about a lot, it's likely that they are 'inside you'. You should remember, however, that sometimes this happens in the unconscious, and when you discover who is inside you, it comes as a revelation.

Ask, 'Is it my mother? My father?'

'My spouse?'

'The culture?'

'A false or limited "I"?'

'Some imagined person who views me critically?'

Once you find who it is you've let in—and you can also find how you have weakened yourself to enable them to come in—politely ask them to leave.

Now call on the Self, God, Guru or Consciousness, and ask that your inner space be expanded and empowered.

Please don't neglect the 'Who is in here?' inquiry. It is a deeply revealing practice.

It should be clear from my exposition how closely related the 'Who is in here?' contemplation is to proxying. Remember these few important points:

- It's never good to internally consider.

- When you internally consider, someone is allowed into your sacred inner space who shouldn't be there (only the Self or God or Guru is allowed there).

- Internal considering compromises your inner freedom and creates contraction and cramp.

- Others enter your inner space (metaphorically, of course) only when you let them by weakening yourself with negative emotion or inappropriate desire.

This explains why it feels so bad to try to force others to do what you want. Here, your inappropriate desire is actually a form of internal considering, and the block and dead weight you feel is that of the other person entering into your inner space with all their resistance and inertia.

Sometimes when we internally consider a person and feel their uncomfortable presence within us, we get angry at them and want to blame them. It would be much better to proxy them because ultimately it is not their fault that they are inside you, but yours.

A NOTE ON ACCEPTING OTHER PEOPLE'S FEELINGS: THE PRACTICE OF TONGLEN

As you pursue Self-inquiry, you become more sensitive and aware of your own and other people's feeling. You risk falling into the disempowering syndrome of excessive fear of other people's negativity. Some people are more afraid of bad feeling than of almost anything else. When they think about the possible loss of a loved one or the failure to achieve some goal, what is most frightening is not so much the event itself, but how that event will make them feel. They think that having such a feeling will annihilate them. But feelings are only feelings. Maybe we are not as great as the ocean-drinking Lord Shiva, but we should be able to interact with others in a robust way. Inquiry should make you less fragile, not more.

In my Learn to Meditate course, I give a meditation technique involving the breath. I ask my students to breathe in, imagining they are drawing energy from outside into themselves. Then they breathe out, imagining they are eliminating toxins and releasing them outside.

This is a good meditation and is in harmony with our usual commonsense view that wants to draw energy into ourselves and send toxicity away from ourselves. The Tibetan Buddhist practice of *tonglen* dramatically reverses this normal state of affairs. *Tonglen* practice asks us to draw all negativity and suffering into ourselves, while sending out love and blessings. This counter-intuitive or anti-egoic practice turns out to be immensely powerful and liberating.

The yogic scriptures declare that human beings are in the thraldom of *raga* and *dvesha*. The ego looks out at the vast world and considers the range of events and possible outcomes that are relevant to it. Some of these outcomes seem favourable and enhance the power, authority or safety of the ego, and others seem unfavourable and threatening.

The ego, therefore, wants certain outcomes (attachment) and wants to avoid other outcomes (aversion). This drama of attachment and aversion creates a tension and increases the suffering of the individual ego. While the ego desperately yearns for favourable outcomes and desperately hates unfavourable ones, the rest of the universe is indifferent. Thus is created a life predicament that is essentially hopeless: no one, as the Buddha noticed, can escape disease, old age and death.

Tonglen practice frees the ego from its bondage to *raga/dvesha* in a single, brilliant stroke. Rather than tensely avoiding the unpleasant, the ego consciously draws it to itself. And rather than tensely seeking the pleasant, it wantonly sends endless blessings to all others. By so doing, it discovers that negative experiences cannot hurt the ego and that the blessings at its command are endless. The ego self stands revealed as the infinite Self of all.

You may have noticed a relationship between *tonglen* and the technique of proxying. Both of these methods compassionately allow the psychic poison experienced in another to enter us. *Tonglen* is even more proactive than proxying, because it actively seeks the negative. In the phone conversation I described in which I was recoiling from Chip, if I were to use *tonglen*, I would actively try to suck all of Chip's poison into me. When you recoil from another person, your being contracts and you become weakened. When you open to another person and embrace them completely, you are powerful and fearless. *Tonglen* may appear like an act of almost lunatic compassion and altruism, but in reality it is one of the most empowering techniques a person can employ for their own welfare. If you do happen to get in trouble doing *tonglen*, you can use proxying to clear the feeling.

CONTEMPLATION:
THE GREAT-HEARTED PRACTICE OF TONGLEN

Think of a person who is difficult for you. Because you find this person's traits or ways disagreeable, you withdraw and recoil from them. In this contemplation, you will go in the opposite direction. As you breathe in, let all of this person's negativity, bad qualities and suffering come into you. With the out-breath, breathe out love, blessings and good wishes to that person. If you watch carefully, I think you will find that the inner energy will be delighted by this practice.

If that is too difficult, try this version. Think of someone you love and with your in-breath, draw in that person's pain and suffering, and with your out-breath, send them love and blessings.

The practice of *tonglen* will make you preposterously strong. You will be able to go anywhere and encounter anything. Fearing nothing, you will engage life unabashedly. You can use an outer form of *tonglen* in the midst of life situations when the tendency to recoil and withdraw arises.

There are two main strategies in life: one is the Vital strategy of seeking the pleasant, seeking fulfilment through objects, and the second is the Solid strategy of avoiding the unpleasant through separation and simplification. A lot of yogis have written about the problems with the first strategy. Endlessly seeking fulfilment of all your desires creates many difficulties. But equally unsatisfactory is the strategy of avoiding the unpleasant. A yogi wants to feel free and open in life, not contracted with fear of engagement. A yogi is a hero, not a coward. The methods of proxying and *tonglen* empower the yogi to avoid recoiling from life, and, rather, face everything with courage.

THE AVIS PROCESS

Another way to deal with other people's feeling is the *Avis Process*, which is a close relative of proxying. Avis is Shiva spelled backwards (Shiva is often spelled 'Siva'). You can use the Avis Process particularly when you are speaking to people who are not 'in the work' (who are not yogis) and who come at you with undigested emotion. Since they are not terribly self-aware and it is not their habit to search for A-Statements, you have to help them with their inquiry without them knowing it. You can ask them questions that point them towards their present experience. You might say things like 'That must have made you very angry' or 'That must be very upsetting'. You make their A-Statements for them: 'Are you feeling upset?' You could offer it like that.

Relationships become unpleasant when negative emotion is present but unacknowledged. In the Avis Process, you strive to have that emotion acknowledged: 'That must make you feel sad' or 'That must make you feel really bad' or 'That must make you feel angry.' Such statements will create a shift. The other person says, 'Yes! I'm *very* angry', and things become more truthful and real.

You can also proxy. In extreme cases, you can proxy inside yourself while you are talking to somebody. Make your statements inwardly while you speak outwardly. This can be amusing. Many Shiva Process practitioners, who deal with work situations and family where inquiry is unknown, use this type of Avis Process a great deal.

The key understanding to hold when you speak with a person who does not practise inquiry is that you must shoulder the responsibility of moving the conversation towards greater reality; that is, towards A-Statements. This helps the other person move towards their personal truth. You will have to do this as self-defence, because the more aware person pays the major price.

Unprocessed feelings seep into a person's outer life from their inner world. In so doing, they create blocks and complexity everywhere. These blocks appear to be external to the person and yet, in reality, find their cause in their own attitude or emotions. They should be returned to that person's inner world to be handled. No amount of juggling outer-world circumstances will get to the basic causes.

The secret of the Avis Process is to 'make the feelings go back inside' the person. In group-inquiry, once the player's feeling has been expressed through A-Statements, it has to go back to them and be processed there. In the Avis Process, it is the responsibility of the yogi to identify the feeling of the other person, articulate it for them, and return it to them.

MAKING THE UNCONSCIOUS CONSCIOUS IN YOUR PRIVATE MEDITATION

All the information we need for spiritual progress is always at hand, but we are not always listening. Train yourself to look and listen to the unconscious; the secret whisper of the Divine. Patanjali describes how to enter a yogic posture, saying (loosely translated): 'Sit in the posture and relax completely. That will put you in touch with the infinite.' Metaphorically, our whole orientation to life is our posture; our *asana*. Through inquiry, we observe the points of tension and relax them in every moment. When we do this effectively, we connect with infinite Consciousness.

You can do this by viewing your whole life as a Shiva Process group. What feedback are you getting? In your personal inquiry, search for the things you have kept hidden from yourself. Ask, for example, questions like 'What message is the universe trying to tell me? Have I heard the same thing two or three times in the past couple of weeks?' Asking such questions allows us to *hear* the voice of God. Information might have come from two or three unrelated sources, as an apparent coincidence. When the same sort of feedback comes from different sources, there is usually a message for you. Such inquiry brings your unconscious to consciousness.

It is particularly profitable to imaginatively allow a person with whom you have a difficult relationship into your inner space. Let that person speak to you and open to their A-Statements. I call this kind of contemplation, 'Listening to your ex-wife' or alternatively, 'Listening to your Guru' or even, 'Listening to your worst enemy'.

Walking the spiritual path for as long as I have, a lot of people have become angry at me, even some great souls. I have gained a lot through letting them speak to me via this contemplation. They would be surprised to know how much I listen to their criticisms. (Yes, I do mean YOU if you are reading this book. And you should let me speak in your meditations, too!) My experience is that far from hurting me, allowing these A-Statements into my meditation fills me with Shakti. The reason for this is that Shakti loves expansion and union, and hates ego and contraction. Therefore, when the ego opens and faces its fears, there are great rewards.

There is really nothing to fear. We resist and fight off this kind of feedback, but that makes us protective and contracted. If we open to it and embrace it, it sets us free. Certainly these people are angry at us, but within their anger, useful messages are hidden. Their anger is frustration because of the carrots we have in our ears, but it translates into Shakti when we remove the carrots. Such methods fill the practitioner with a strange joy. The Shakti *loves* it when you look at your unconscious—*loves* it—because you are merging in Consciousness and transcending the ego.

CONVERSATIONS WITH SHIVA

We can also communicate with others whom are no longer present to us. Every relationship and situation in your life is nothing but a collection of *matrikas*, spoken and unspoken, blocked or flowing. This whole universe is nothing but Shiva's word play. If that's the case, getting to stillness in meditation won't put an end to life's difficulties any more than going to sleep at night means that the world will not rise up again the next morning. Along with going into the silence, you have to learn how to bring all the systems of *matrika* to peace and harmony.

When people leave your outer world by moving away or by death, they're still reachable through the inner world. Every part of the universe, past, present or future, is accessible in the inner world. Only a small fragment is accessible through the outer world. Thus, inner speech is even more powerful than verbalisation. You can sort out your relations with departed ones, with dead relatives, with people who are far away, and with people with whom you have unresolved or unfinished conversations.

Inwardly, tell your dead father what you've always needed to tell him. In some way or some realm he will hear you. As you do this, watch the movement of feeling within yourself. When you move from contraction and suffering to expansion and love, understand that you are bringing your *matrikas* into equilibrium. I have no doubt that sitting in your room, speaking to people in your inner world, you can resolve the most profound issues of your life.

CONTEMPLATION: TALKING TO A DEAD RELATIVE

There's likely to be something incomplete in your relationship with a departed person. Imagining them in front of you, say what needs to be said. As before, pay attention to the movement of feeling. As needed, you can proxy them. Always try to end by bringing things into harmony. Let them speak to you.

And, of course, you can speak to the higher power, to God, within yourself. You should 'make yourself known at the court of the king'. Tell universal Consciousness exactly what you want and what you fear. Ask inwardly for exactly what you want without being timid or politically correct. I call this process 'conversations with Shiva'. Once you've made yourself known to the highest, to the court of last resort, you can then let it go and surrender to God's will.

CONTEMPLATION: TELL SHIVA WHAT YOU WANT

Look within and focus on the highest principle: Shiva, Jesus, Krishna, the Guru, the Self, higher Consciousness. Now, frankly and unembarrassedly, ask for exactly what you want. Don't pull your punches. Make sure you include what you don't want. While you do this, watch carefully for the shifts in feeling, and let those be your guide. Let Shiva speak to you.

SPECIALISED SHIVA PROCESS GROUPS

In addition to Proxying and Avis Processing, a number of specialised inquiry groups are effective under specific conditions.

- *Designer Groups* are tailored to deal with an issue or a person:

The members of such a group are hand-picked, either for their connection to the person involved, or their expertise or objectivity vis-à-vis the issue involved. You might have a designer group about Fred's drinking problem, which would include members of his family and friends and also people with experience in the area of alcoholism (psychologists, recovering alcoholics and so on). Or, you might have a designer group to settle a dispute over a car between Chip and Ugrasena. The members of this group would probably be fair-minded business people.

- *Area of Life Groups* divide into the categories of:

  - Health and body

  - Career, work and money

  - Relationships (couple groups are a subclass)

  - Spirituality.

The leader of an area of life group should be someone who successfully navigates the area concerned.

- *Task-Oriented Groups* usually arise in the workplace:

A discussion of the task at hand happens in the normal way, but Shiva Process methods are brought in as the need arises; that is, when a block comes up. Such a group presupposes familiarity with Shiva Process method. This type of group is sometimes called a 'Shiva Process conversation' because it flows in an unstructured way, except when the discipline needs to be applied.

Meetings in the ashram here all take the form of a Shiva Process conversation in that inquiry might break out any time that second force arises. Inquiry can discover the core issues and avoid running roughshod over a minority point of view that may have something valuable to add.

To begin a task-oriented group, the leader conducts a different sort of guided meditation than usual. Let's say the staff and management of a cafe come together to deal with work-related issues. The leader says, 'Let's contemplate the cafe. Let's think about the food ... the service ... the coffee ...the decor ...the menu ... the staff ... the management and so on. Note the areas of tension or concern'. After such a meditation, play proceeds in the normal way with each participant giving their report.

It should be noted that a second approach to a task-oriented group is to simply bring together the relevant people for a normal Shiva Process. The idea here is that the Shiva Process conducted among them will have the byproduct of improving the work situation, and that, where necessary, work issues will probably arise spontaneously anyway.

- *Solid, Vital and Peculiar Groups* divide into like types:

The larger group splits into three smaller groups. Solid types work with others of the same type, and similarly for Vital and Peculiar types. Or groups can form according to where the life current appears at the time: the head, the navel or the heart.

- *Intellectual Shiva Process Groups* focus on ideas:

There are always a few meditators in my classes who tell me they can't get in touch with feeling in any of their centres. They're usually Solids or Vitals. Finding an appropriate method for such people is far better than trying to change them. One of the solutions which works for Solid practitioners is the intellectual Shiva Process group. Here, ideas are offered as feedback, and the player evaluates them according to whether they have more or less energy, or more or less light.

There could also be a Vital Shiva Process group in which possible actions are offered and evaluated according to how empowering they feel. The personal preferences of group leaders will colour the way they lead the group. One person is more comfortable with ideas, one person is more comfortable with feelings. To an extreme Peculiar, groups led by an extreme Solid may always seem like an intellectual Shiva Process, and the reverse is also true.

THE BIG GAME

The most powerful and effective method of group-inquiry is *The Big Game*. When a spiritual crisis is at hand, when a big block or blind spot needs to be dealt with, it is time to employ The Big Game. When ordinary methods do not work and the group encounters a recurrent block, The Big Game increases the energy of inquiry. It is like shifting into overdrive.

Ordinarily, The Big Game is organised in advance, with the player's knowledge and consent. A player plays as usual—people ask questions, they make statements and so on, but at a certain point, that player is asked to leave the room. The group discusses the person, seeking to *discover what Consciousness wants to say to the player*. This might sound like your worst nightmare—being gossiped about behind your back! It is actually not that: The Big Game is a compassionate and powerful feedback device.

Why does the player have to leave the room? Notice that in ordinary life there are people to whom you can't say certain things. It becomes easier to gossip about them in their absence and, regrettably or not, this happens all the time. When a person leaves the room to play The Big Game, it is acknowledged that there is a block in communication. Whatever the group has to say to that person may be raw and undigested, creating defensiveness in the player. In the player's absence, the group takes time to sift through matters to find out what its real message is and formulate a kind way to get the information home, to speak to the player's listening.

The leader collects data from the group, writing down ideas on a whiteboard. The leader's responsibility is to deliver the information to the player when they return in such a way that truth and kindness are balanced, and any personal elements and judgments are weeded out. If, for example, one of the participants has malice for the player and gives their input in that way, that part of it has to be eliminated while constructive elements are retained. Another person has their own emotional reaction to the process and that also should be discarded as irrelevant to the player.

The leader must listen carefully to hear what *Consciousness* wants to say. Consciousness speaks through people. It speaks through all the individuals. If you can eliminate the ego and personal factors, you can discover what Consciousness is saying. If the leader has doubts, it is worth checking their intuition with the group. Everyone in the group should be satisfied with the conclusions of the group. Each person should agree with the group finding and not suppress their real opinion. If one or two are not in agreement, that must be told to the player when they return (without, of course, saying who thinks what).

When the group reaches agreement, or as much agreement as is possible, the player returns and the leader tells the player what Consciousness (the group) wants said. The leader, even during this part of the process, should confirm things with the group.

Leading The Big Game is a challenge. The leader has to tune in to hear the message of the Divine *through* and *behind* the feedback of individuals. The solutions are always there, but may be hidden. Players who are prepared to listen to what Consciousness—and not an individual—is saying to them will receive a tremendous blessing. It offers something really powerful to work with. It exposes what is hiding in the unconscious and therefore blocking their ability to move forward in life and in self-knowledge.

The Big Game is the best medicine for your unconscious. It is like looking into the mirror of Consciousness and asking, 'What does God want to tell me?' The Big Game generates an answer. Almost everyone has a stuck point in one or another area of their life, and The Big Game is *hathapaka*; a sudden and jolting method of growth.

The Big Game should always include at least one D-Statement, an 'action-command', as homework. Doing the homework puts the insights of The Big Game into concrete effect in the person's life. No one should play The Big Game if they are not prepared to take on the instructions of the group. That doesn't mean the player has to passively accept them. They are entitled to speak up and argue if they like, though that could lead to further blocks. But playing The Big Game implies an agreement to abide by the group's directives. More than one Big Game has ended with the group distilling all the information into just one action statement, like 'You should have lunch with your mother'. Mysteriously, in those cases, that is the only thing that the group wants to say, and mysteriously also, that homework has a powerful effect.

LEADING GROUP-INQUIRY

As the leader in The Big Game has the responsibility of searching for what Consciousness wants to tell the player, so too does the leader in regular group-inquiry. The leader is not an all-knowing expert who intuitively knows what's good for you and tells it to you in no uncertain terms. Rather, they are a servant of Consciousness and should scrupulously look for what Consciousness itself, and not they personally, wants to say. In fact, it's a relief for the leader, who doesn't have to be a genius or a clairvoyant, but can make use of the talents and intuition of others in the group. It's a good sign if the leader is occasionally surprised by what happens in the group and also discovers that their own opinions and values are sometimes confronted. This proves that a higher power than the leader's ego and opinion is at work.

One day, I will write a handbook for Shiva Process leaders, but I'll limit myself here to a few remarks. At the time of this writing, I have designated group leaders after they've worked with me for a long time and I've watched their work closely. I'm in the process of creating a more formal training.

As we saw regarding specialised groups, different leaders inevitably have different leadership styles. Some emphasise story more and some less. Whether the leader is a Solid, a Vital or a Peculiar also affects the group. It's appropriate also to take advantage of the unique skills or perspective of the leader.

Ma Devi's training, for example, in Gestalt therapy sometimes gives groups led by her such a singular quality that we call it the *Shakti Process*. The Shakti Process is therapeutic in its approach. It focuses on the personal, unconscious or conscious hurt that needs to be released. Tearing thoughts and the feelings associated with the hurt are explored. This works particularly well for people suffering from addictions, stuck in negative thinking or with behaviour patterns that block love. Because of her connection to and awareness of the spiritual energy, it remains Shiva Process, but, surely, it's near the borderline between Shiva Process and Gestalt.

You can see from this example that the Shiva Process tolerates a wide range of styles and flavours, recognising that they are all different permutations of Consciousness. After all, Consciousness contains the infinite manifestation of the universe. But what is indispensable is that the leader be dedicated to the process and to the present moment, and have a sense that the mutual undertaking is sacred, which is not to say humourless.

When I lead a group, I feel that, mystically, the answers are held somewhere in the collective, not just in my perception. Consciousness always knows everything. What I cannot see, someone else can see from their own perspective. Sitting in a circle is like viewing a statue from 360 degrees. Each angle discloses something new and unique. Each person should be respectfully regarded as holding a piece of the total vision, even when they can't articulate it properly.

Perhaps in writing about the principles of group-inquiry, I've made it sound like a logical and practical progression from darkness to light. I wish it were true! More frequently, a Shiva Process group is like a journey through a complex landscape without a map. There are moments of great clarity and insight, but also moments of confusion and obscurity. There is nothing wrong with that. What would be wrong is for the leader to keep up a pretence that everything is always clear and under control. When things are murky, the leader should ask questions like 'What's happening now? Has the energy gone up or down? Have we lost the thread? Have we lost presence? Do things seem murky?' thus bringing attention to the present situation. The fall-back position is expressed in the phrase: 'Say what is so.' If you feel confused in the middle of a group, a good place to go is to say, 'I'm confused'. Take refuge in present reality.

The leader should be in a clear and impersonal space. Sometimes, however, the flow of the group will elicit a personal reaction from the leader. The leader then has to become a player, giving the leadership, at least temporarily, to another.

The leader keeps the movement of the group flowing and also holds the discipline of the group. The leader decides when the play has to move from, for example, A-Statements to B-Statements, or one player to another. The leader encourages those who are silent to participate more fully and also encourages those who talk endlessly to discipline their speech. The leader has to keep an appropriate balance between story and feeling. In my own practice, I am a minimalist. I'm likely to move on once there is any shift at all.

QUESTIONS AND ANSWERS

FINDING THE SEED

Question: I like your analogy of the detective story. Inquiry is so interesting and it seems that I always come up with surprising things; things I never imagined were there.

Swamiji: Yes, that's part of my delight, too—like solving a chess puzzle. One of the *Shiva Sutras* says, *Bijavadhanam:* 'Focus on the seed.' To my mind, this has two meanings. The perhaps more profound one is to take 'seed' to be the Self, therefore Consciousness is always at the centre of everything. The author of the *Shiva Sutras* is thus telling us to always remember the Self under all circumstances of life.

The other meaning is perhaps less profound, but it might be more interesting! In this interpretation, seed has to do with emotion or intention. Everything we do has some underlying feeling or motive, and that completely affects the results, the outcome and our experience. Thus, intelligent meditators are as keen to know their own motives as they are to know the motives of others. We also eat the fruit of the seed that we plant. It only makes good sense to know what that seed is. As the song says, 'Plant a carrot, Get a carrot, Not a Brussels sprout'. It's good to know the seed.

WHERE TO BEGIN

Question: Are you suggesting that we begin every session of group-inquiry with the opening statements?

Swamiji: No. I do suggest that you always begin with the guided meditation. The opening statements are optional. Their purpose is to focus awareness on the task at hand and centre it in Consciousness. If you did it every time, it could become too mechanical. One idea is to use the opening statements in the same way, I'm told, that some 12-

step programs use the steps—the leader could pick one out for emphasis and comment on it.

Another method is to begin the guided meditation by first invoking higher Consciousness. You could call on the Guru, God, Shakti or qualities like health, wisdom and love. You might also, at the same time, renounce obstacles like ego, attachment and aversion, opinions, fear, anger and ignorance. Patanjali mentions two methods: a positive one, *abhyasa*, spiritual effort or practice; and a negative one, *vairagya*, a letting go. By embracing the higher qualities and letting go of the lower ones, you clear the deck for an effective group process. Let your intuition lead you here. As I say, the only thing I insist on is the guided meditation. The purpose of the opening statements is to bring everyone present to the task at hand.

GOING DEEPER

Question: Can the inquiry become stale and mechanical when people know each other too well?

Swamiji: Yes, that can happen, and it happens in marriage relationships as well. Nonetheless, there are always ways to press the refresh button and go deeper and bring in more energy. Since the Self is dynamism itself, stagnations only amount to a temporary falling asleep. The antidote to stagnation is upping the truth ante of the group. Remember, the leader can ask for more truth, and the group members can resolve to bring more truth content to their play. That will enliven things quickly.

Related to this, but in the opposite direction, it sometimes happens that members of a group feel they have 'bonded' and are therefore reluctant to take on new members. This kind of bonding can be good if it creates more trust, but it has the danger of turning the group into a little cult, which serves the ego more than the impersonal Self.

THE MYSTERY OF PROXYING

Question: You mentioned that you proxied an art gallery. That really got my attention. Could you say something more about that?

Swamiji: Every place has its own atmosphere. The atmosphere isn't in the bricks and stones, but resides in the thoughts and feelings that have clustered around the location. For that reason, holy sites, places of pilgrimage, have a spiritual charge. And certain homes have a distinct feeling of sadness or joy, as the case may be. In a world of Consciousness, everything is alive and has its own vibration and its own feeling.

One of the most remarkable proxyings I ever did was the Dog Shiva Process. One of my students is a vet, and a number of years ago she brought four or five dog owners and their dogs and we did a Shiva Process; the owners making statements for the dogs. It was quite mysterious and humorous, but I will swear to you the dogs had shifts. Then again, so did the owners. Well, why not, isn't the dog just an extension of the owner's subtle body? As the atmosphere in the room changed, the dogs became much more relaxed and friendly. The owners did, too. It was all hilarious and exhilarating.

MAKING THE LEAP TO GROUP-INQUIRY

Question: I enjoy doing personal inquiry but I find that I'm quite terrified of group-inquiry. Should I simply continue with the personal inquiry or make a leap into the fire?

Swamiji: It's not as scary as all that. Group-inquiry is, in fact, a compassionate method. But having said that, there is definitely an intensification. It feels like you are playing for higher stakes. Although the premise of group-inquiry is goodwill, it also requires fearlessness.

I have pointed out that the Buddhist practices of *chod* and *tonglen* affront the ego. The ego always wants to be safe and dominant. These practices turn the tables on the ego and let the 'worst' happen. They even invite the worst to happen. In New York, we used to ask, first of all, 'What's the worst-case scenario?' We wanted to know what the worst outcome was before we embarked on anything. Wisdom tells us that embodied existence is already the worst-case scenario.

The service inherent in group process involves sacrifice and is risky from the ego's point of view, but, as I have said, it is a risk that has great rewards. And spiritually, we have to pay less attention to the demands of the ego as we walk the path.

I hope I have reassured rather than scared you. Truly, there is nothing to be afraid of. By the rules of the Shiva Process, if you feel scared, you should just say, 'I feel scared', and everyone else will say, 'That's a good statement'. See how easy it is?

INQUIRY FOR THE BODY

Question: I have undiagnosable chest pains, which I think are a weakness in my heart. No doctor has found the problem. Can inquiry be helpful?

Swamiji: Yes it can. We hold unconscious attitudes towards parts of our body. It's good to make these attitudes conscious, and then work on them. Do an inquiry on your relationship with your heart. Ask yourself, 'What do I feel about my heart?' You may discover that you think of it as weak and have done so all your life. Notice that it may actually be weak, or it may not be weak at all, although you think it is.

Proxy your heart. Say, 'I am my heart and I feel weak. I am my heart and I'm overworked. I am my heart and I want more oxygen'. In this way, get close to your unconscious thoughts about your heart. Once you've done that, you can do a healing meditation. Breathe strength, oxygen, vitality into your heart. I think you get the idea. Whatever organ or part of the body you have a problem with, investigate, inquire and treat it by means of meditation. Of course, I'm not suggesting that you shouldn't pursue medical options. Do so. On the other hand, we hold a surprising number of wrong attitudes that give us trouble and should be ferreted out.

Question: In recent years, I have had a lot of physical problems. Could you talk more about using inquiry in the area of body and health?

Swamiji: There is no fundamental difference in method, no matter what area of life we are investigating. Inquiry should be direct and to the point, moving closer and closer to the truth. As you get closer to the truth, your inquiry releases energy. With regard to health, you might ask yourself where you feel pain or weakness in your body. When you find significant areas, inquire into the cause. Is it related to diet, substance abuse, negative emotion and so on? Ask what you need to do. You may get an answer like 'Change your diet' or 'See a doctor or acupuncturist'. The main thing here is to confront the sensations directly. Out of that confrontation, information will come. As I've mentioned, remarkable results come from specialised group-inquiry— attending a group that focuses on health issues would be worthwhile.

You can call on your immune system to stand up and defend yourself. You can call on the healing power of the Divine; you can send love and energy to various organs or areas of the body. You can try saying the word 'health' on the in-breath and dispelling toxicity on the out-breath. Use your imagination and always look for the upward shift. Don't forget that universal Shakti or *prana* is the greatest healing force. *Prana* contains all the vitamins and proteins in the universe. All animals and plants depend on *prana* for their lives. How powerful, then, must *prana* be?

Now, I'll tell you the greatest healing meditation I know. Imagine that God has created the perfect medicine for your condition, knowing exactly what's wrong with you and what you need. This medicine is healing, nutritious, life-positive and full of life force. Now imagine that medicine is mixed with your breath, and when you breathe in, you are breathing that medicine in and it fills your body with its perfectly intelligent healing power. Some of you may prefer to use the out-breath for this exercise, but either way, I think you will have good results.

I don't want you to get the idea that I am a Christian Scientist. No, you should consult medical practitioners, but along with that, you can use inquiry in the area of health.

ASKING FOR WHAT YOU WANT

Question: I have resistance to your instruction to pray for what I want. Sometimes I feel that what I want is inappropriate, and even disgusting. How can I deal with this?

Swamiji: Yes, I do tell people to pray for what they want and not for what they think they *should* want. In golf, the secret is to get your full weight behind your swing. Everything should be moving together in the same direction. In a bad swing, different parts go in opposite directions, dissipating energy. You can only achieve something important through complete mental, emotional and volitional integration; the marriage of head and heart. If your head and heart are going in opposite directions, then you have a divided self.

Praying for what you want is not arrogance, but actually a kind of humility. It's making an A-Statement, which puts you into an undivided space. Even if what you want is 'disgusting', it's good to admit it. Admit it in the privacy of your prayer. Once you admit it to yourself, it won't be working unconsciously within you, and you will give up inappropriate desires very naturally.

A *Siddha* is one who is undivided. There is an old story from the Zen tradition about a blind man who lived near a master who had just died. He told a friend, 'I judge character by the sound of people's voices. When someone congratulates somebody, I hear a secret tone of envy. When another offers condolence, I hear a hint of pleasure at another's pain. Only the master had no such undertone. When he expressed happiness, I heard nothing but happiness, and when he expressed sorrow, I heard nothing but sorrow'.

Try this meditation:

CONTEMPLATION: ALIGNING HEAD AND HEART

Define and acknowledge where you are conflicted or uncertain. Try to align your heart and your mind. If you are caught between alternatives and you can't overcome them, it is possible to get your weight behind something like 'I'd like to reach certainty in this issue'. You can now pray for certainty with an undivided heart.

SEEPING FEELING

Question: In inquiry groups I've attended, it's been hard sometimes to end the telling of the story and begin the process of feedback. Could you comment on that?

Swamiji: If you do group-inquiry with experienced people, what happens is that someone suddenly says, 'I have feedback' and then feedback begins. What actually happens is they're responding to the player's feeling seeping into the room. When that feeling seeps sufficiently into the room, it has to be given back to the player by means of feedback. There has to be a little bit of seepage so the group contacts the issue, but ultimately the player has to process it within.

This is why we find people unpleasant. Their unprocessed feeling seeps into us and we feel gagged or paralysed by it. It's necessary for us to find a way to process that feeling by sending it back to them via either the Avis Process or proxying it, as I did with Chip. Otherwise, we will run screaming from the room, feeling angry at the perpetrator.

When unprocessed feeling seeps into us, it is confusing. It's important the group begins feedback at the right time or else the player's story will contaminate the group process and make it stupid.

INFINITE HAPPINESS

Question: Sometimes I notice in group-inquiry that I feel better but someone else feels worse, or I feel worse and someone else feels better. I wonder if there is a certain amount of happiness and a certain amount of misery and it just travels around the group.

Swamiji: No, no, no! You remind me of one of Samuel Beckett's characters who used to say that the 'quantum of wantum cannot vary'. I understand why you think like that, but that is material thinking, thinking from a sense of limitation. It is the same kind of thinking that says, 'The sun is cooling down and the earth's petroleum resources are drying up'. Maybe the earth's petroleum resources are limited, but Consciousness is infinite. Happiness and joy can be expanded infinitely.

There is, however, an issue about coming away with residual or negative feelings or having a downward shift. It happens, and there are methods for dealing with it, such as using the closing statements, although we may not always apply them properly. In the flow of conversation and inquiry, these things happen. Perhaps it signifies we have had a failure in our Shiva Process technique, but it might be more profitable to regard such things as presenting an opportunity for further growth. You should not worry so much about contaminating others, or being contaminated yourself, that you don't engage in inquiry freely.

LEADING A GROUP

Question: I've led my fair share of inquiry groups and I find that it works best for me if there's an assistant leader. Any comments?

Swamiji: Yes, I find that having an assistant leader is an excellent idea, although you can do groups on your own if there's no one appropriate at hand. An assistant is particularly useful when something arises in the group that engages the leader. When the leader has to play, they cannot also lead. The leader can pass leadership of the group to the assistant during their own play, and then take it back at the end.

When I'm running a group with an assistant, I'll make use of the assistant by asking them for input at various times. For example, when it's time to designate the first player, I'll ask the assistant to name three people that need to play. An assistant is useful to provide another point of view.

Question: When leading groups on a theme like workplace or relationships, play often centres around the issue of choosing between two alternatives. Do you have any tips to handle this?

Swamiji: The ancient texts unanimously say that doubt is one of the great spiritual impediments. What is doubt but being caught between alternatives? One text says doubt is 'maybe this, maybe that'. When you're saying, 'maybe this, maybe that', you're not going anywhere, you are just sitting with 'maybe this, maybe that'. Thus, doubt paralyses you.

When I'm in that situation, I sometimes call for the separation of the two alternatives. I ask the player to fully explore each alternative by itself as though that were the one that was fully accepted. After doing that, I'll have the group give feedback and so on as normal. Then I'll ask the player to do exactly the same with the other alternative. If there are three possibilities, we do it three times. This way, we move past the stuck point and create possibilities under each alternative. Remarkably, the 'right choice' frequently emerges because it is much more filled with life and good energy than the other options.

You can try this in your group. Let's imagine that in an infinite universe, there are infinite you's making infinite choices. In some universes, you choose 'A' and in others you choose 'not A'. You can probably live with either of them, though one might be better. But it's essential to choose.

This hints at two of the goals of a group process: clarification and action. The group leader, or any member of the group, provides an intellectual service by defining what the real alternatives are, by looking with clarity at the emotional morass that has been presented. Once the player is clear about alternatives (rather than getting lost in bewailing their cruel fate), action becomes possible.

PERSONALITY TYPES AND THE PROCESS

Question: It's been my experience that Solids and Peculiars approach the Shiva Process differently, and maybe they have different needs. Could you comment on that?

Swamiji: First of all, you'd have to say that the Shiva Process is a Solid mechanism for dealing with emotion. It doesn't allow negative emotion to expand and be indulged, but creates a discipline wherein we take the negative emotions to their source. On the other hand, there are many Peculiar elements to the group process. Feedback is one such Peculiar feature since it allows such a wide and relatively uncensored range of possibilities.

Peculiars get into trouble by milking the story for all it's worth. An underlying Peculiar A-Statement might be 'I've been misunderstood and hurt and I can prove it', hence the Peculiar wants to tell you their story. Peculiars just love to tell their story. As the story is told, the feeling exudes into the room unpleasantly. The discipline of Shiva Process, in the case of the Peculiar, requires that the story gets limited and the feeling is dealt with directly.

The opposite is true for a Solid. Solids are like the characters played by Gary Cooper; silent and inexpressive. It's hard to get the story from them because story brings up feeling. If I were to cite a typical underlying Solid A-Statement, it might be something like 'My feelings are small and insignificant and what happens to me is not terribly important, and I want to remain calm'. The discipline for a Solid, then, is for them to bring out more story, and with it, the genuine feeling.

THE MYSTICAL ELEMENT

Question: Would you say you have a mystical sense of the Shiva Process group?

Swamiji: Yes, Consciousness is the most mysterious of all things. How do we know, perceive, think, love and remember? For that matter, how do we speak and understand? How is it that you and I can create sentences on the fly and they fall into place and even communicate meaning to another without rehearsing them? How can this be? It's astounding, isn't it? And how can it be that I'm present, alive and aware in this precise moment of time surrounded by an infinite expanse before and an infinite expanse after?

And there's more. I'm convinced that God as the Self or universal Consciousness is not far away at all, but in fact extremely close, though behind a veil. Remember the movie *Ghost?* The soul of the departed lover wanted to communicate with the living partner, but had no instrument to do it until he found the Whoopi Goldberg character. In the same way, God is close at hand and wants to communicate with each of us. That communication is blocked by personal and egoic elements which make us unconscious of parts of our psyche. The Shiva Process group creates conditions in which God can speak, or perhaps more accurately, conditions in which we can hear Him.

EXPANDING THE ENERGY

Question: How would you express the essence of Shiva Process?

Swamiji: Inquiry can be boiled down to three questions. The first is 'What's going on here?' The second is 'What's really going on here?' The third is 'What's really, really going on here?' If you grasp that in the right way, you will understand inquiry.

The Shiva Process group-inquiry is all about retaining and expanding energy. Because we are often irresponsible in our thoughts and communications, we dissipate energy through negative emotion and self-indulgence. We leak energy. A lot of people talk themselves down as they tell you about themselves. Even though they feel increasingly worse as they continue talking, something compels them to go on. In fact, they are not fully aware of what they are doing to themselves.

Group-inquiry disciplines this tendency. For example, as the person speaks about an issue, the feeling comes into the room. At a certain point, the group turns to feedback, which turns the feeling back towards the person. It puts the story back inside where the feeling belongs, and the person becomes responsible for what they are producing. With the aid of feedback, the person begins to process their feeling, and by B- and G-Statements, uplifts it. The group-inquiry method is simply a disciplined conversation. It aims at upliftment and expansion, overcoming the bad habits that dissipate our energy and plunge us into misery.

Yogis know that their happiness or unhappiness is their own manifestation based on their use of inner and outer language. Group-inquiry makes us become more aware and intelligent about our manifestation and teaches us to take control of it.

SUMMARY

- Group work may be better understood via a series of metaphors: the vision quest; the electrical current; the mirror; the detective story; the movement from gross to subtle; the sacred fire.

- Truth and love offered into Consciousness make the fire of awareness blaze brighter.

- Opening statements hone the group's attention and reaffirm its purpose.

- Closing questions examine the results and make them conscious.

- Proxying is processing someone else as if in their shoes.

- External considering is speaking to people where they're at.

- Internal considering is the tendency to see ourselves negatively as though through others' eyes.

- The practice of *tonglen* is a radical form of proxying.

- Listening to your ex-wife and your worst enemy in your meditation helps make the unconscious conscious.

- Past, present and future are accessible through the inner world.

- You can speak to anyone, dead or alive, human or divine, in your inner world.

- The Avis Process uses indirect means to point others towards their present experience.

- Shiva Process groups may be tailored to an issue, person, area of life, task, personality type or ideas.

- The Big Game is the most powerful way to hear what Consciousness wants to tell you.

- The group leader is a servant of Consciousness.

- The Shakti Process works on a player's recurring issue or stuck point.

- It is important to know your own motives in the group and in general.

- An assistant leader is useful in group-inquiry to provide another point of view.

- The right choice is marked by good energy.

- You can proxy parts of the body, institutions, nations and animals.

- Praying for what you want is not arrogance but is making an A-Statement.

- In group-inquiry, it is important to begin feedback at the right time or else the player's feeling may contaminate the process.

- Group-inquiry creates conditions in which we can hear God speak.

- The essence of the Shiva Process is to retain and expand energy.

PART III
THREE MOVEMENTS

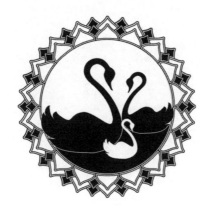

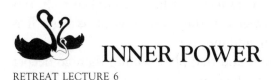 **INNER POWER**

> *This, indeed, is Shiva. Indeed, this too is Shiva. Indeed, this*
> *too is Shiva. Indeed, this too is Shiva. This is my teaching. This*
> *is my teaching. This is my teaching. This is my teaching.*
>
> **Guru Gita**

> *Everything is possible.*
>
> **Anandamayi Ma**

I'VE FINISHED MY discussion of group-inquiry. This chapter is based on a talk I gave at the retreat's culminating Intensive program. It's a summary of everything that has been said, and contains a different paradigm through which inquiry can be viewed.

I like to begin every program remembering my Guru, Baba Muktananda, who would begin every talk he gave by saying, *Subko bare sammane ki sath premse hardik swagat:* 'With great respect and love, I welcome you all with all my heart.' Every night, he would explain that true spirituality is not about practices and difficult and complex philosophies, but is simply about welcoming another person with love and respect. If we can do that much, then true spirituality is ours. We may know the scriptures and do a lot of yogic practice, but if we are not open and loving to others, and don't treat them with respect and kindness, then we are only a sham. To welcome another with love and respect—that is the essence of it.

At the same time, I must also give my own message because I am afraid that if I don't, the sky might fall or the earth might implode.

So, my message is this: within every person there is a great power and a great potential. Some call it the *kundalini shakti* and some call it the inner Self. It is the divine Consciousness within each of us. When we become aware of it, when we awaken it, when we awaken to it, our life is transformed. This power is within every one of us here. It is within you and you and you, and me also.

If you know that power and that place within, then go deeper into it. The more you know it, the more meaning and joy your life will have. If you don't know that power and place within yourself, I say to you, wake up to your true nature! Life is not only the endless whirl of mundane concerns and petty pleasures. Seek the place of inner power and you will surely find it. The fact is that, since you are here today or reading this, you have an interest in the Self and that means you are close to awakening.

The other day, someone gave me something from a sacred text called *New Idea* [a women's magazine]. It says:

> Thinking sad thoughts can make you ill, new research has found. Human subjects were asked to think happy or sad thoughts and be monitored for brain activity. They were given flu shots and those who showed negative brain activity were shown to have the weakest immune system over six months. 'Emotions play an important role in modulating bodily systems that influence health', says Richard Davidson, a distinguished US neuroscientist.

Isn't that good? I like to imagine the subjects assiduously thinking happy or sad thoughts. Would that it were so easy to think happy thoughts! Us yogis would be out of business.

There is some knowledge of A- and B-Statements here. While, undoubtedly, people who feel good can fall ill, there certainly is a strong link between our physical health and our inner state—our mental state.

Spanda Karikas is one of the great texts of Kashmir Shaivism; probably my favourite text. It is a collection of short verses expounding Shaivite ideas. The scriptural and Shaivite roots of the Self-inquiry we do, the Shiva Process, are in that text. Here is where *Spanda Karikas* agrees with *New Idea*.

Glanir vilunthika dehe tasyashchchajnanataha shritihi
Tadunmesha-viluptam chet kutaha sa syad ahetuka

Just as a plunderer carries away the valuables of the house, even so depression saps away the vitality of the body. This depression proceeds from ignorance. If that ignorance disappears by [the expansion of knowledge of the Self] ... how can that depression last in the absence of its cause?

Have you ever suffered a burglary in your house? It is a terrible shock—you feel violated and drained of energy. In the same way, depression saps the vitality of the body. It is a kind of theft. The yogis have always known that when you have a negative flow of thoughts, an abundance of tearing thoughts, everything is depressed—your immune system, everything. And it shows up when you investigate it through inquiry.

But here is something new: *Spanda Karikas* says, 'This depression proceeds from ignorance'. *New Idea* says, when you think happy thoughts, your immune system grows stronger. But Shaivism's insight, that ignorance causes depression, is important. If, as the scriptures say, we are divine beings, it's our tearing thoughts that diminish us. Believing these tearing thoughts is ignorance. In my pre-yoga days, I believed my tearing thoughts. Meditation and inquiry showed me that they were simply wrong. It was a healing knowledge.

The *Spanda Karikas* says, 'If that ignorance disappears by *unmesha*, how can that depression last in the absence of its cause?' *Unmesha* refers to the upward shift of energy; the upward flow. When we experience it, then depression and ignorance leave us. We connect with the inner power. The problem here is that our negative thought-forms separate us from the inner power. Our yoga, our spirituality, must connect us to that inner power. That is what it is all about; nothing more and nothing less.

I would add this to what *New Idea* says: there is a place within us that is perfect and serene. It can be known. We can connect with it. The main barrier to it is our negative train of thought. Through inner practice we can transcend that negative train of thought, or understand it profoundly and shift it. Either method returns us to the Self.

The Self is always present. The Self is always present. The Self is always present. (In India, when you want your students to really 'get' something, you repeat it three times. It is Indian verbal italics.) The negative tendency of thought is well established in us by birth trauma, by early abuse, by those naughty parents of ours. Hindu philosophy would add to our list of causes countless lifetimes of bad thinking and bad living. This indicates how strong our negative patterns are. Have you noticed how strong the negative strain is—the tearing thoughts—how strong and persistent they are? It sounds right that such persistence is the result of lifetimes of bad tendencies.

Self-inquiry is, as they say now, a 24/7 kind of thing. It is ongoing. It is about awareness. My Buddhist teacher, Sri Goenka, used to say, in a voice like the actor Peter Lorre, 'Go into the feeling throughout the body, feel the feelings throughout the body. It is all *anitya*. It is all illusion, it is non-existent. Run the mind through the body. Be aware. Be aware. Be aware!' All the great sages exhort us in this way.

I am going to discuss inquiry once again, but from a slightly different perspective. Inquiry has three movements to it. They are:

- Investigation
- Recognition
- Upliftment and Transformation

INVESTIGATION

Investigation is the first step and the prerequisite here is not to be afraid of what is inside you. People sometimes tell me, 'I am terrified to know what is in me' as though there were an axe-murderer in there. Well, perhaps there is an axe-murderer in there, but we know now that inside the axe-murderer is the Self.

Our *fundamental* nature is the Self—peace, truth and love. Yes, it can be distorted. Yes, every monster in history has gone off in hideous ways; it can't be denied. But the essence is always there, however twisted the personality. It is essential to know that our fundamental nature is pure. We don't have to be afraid to go inside. In fact, if discovered, that axe-murderer can be diffused by inquiry. It is always better to know what is going on inside than not to know. It does take courage and a certain amount of enlightenment to even be interested in meditation, inquiry and the spiritual process. So, I congratulate us!

Investigation has two aspects. One is observation, which is simply looking; paying attention to what *is*. The second is inquiry, which is asking questions. As mentioned earlier, I prefer 'what' to 'why'. My version of the primary spiritual question, the question all great beings have asked, is: 'What's going on here?' This is the same question that science asks. In fact, the same question is asked in many fields. If you are a sociologist, a psychologist, a chemist, a weatherman or a chess player, the first question is always, 'What's going on here?'

While the question is the same, the difference lies in the object under investigation. In spirituality, the object is the Self. Paradoxically, it is said that the Self can never be an object. Vedanta says that you can never make the Self an object; you can only say what the Self is *not*. In inquiry, we investigate the blocks that separate us from the Self. While the Self cannot be an object of investigation, the investigator can know the Self as the subject, as the experience of subjectivity.

INQUIRY: WHAT'S GOING ON HERE?

Close your eyes and ask the question, 'What's going on here?' More likely than not, several different things are going on. Thoughts are happening. You may have a good feeling, be excited, have a sense of anticipation, or you may have a negative feeling. You may be carrying something from an encounter earlier today. These are all valid answers to 'What's going on here?' In real inquiry, you try to find out what is so; you don't paste over it and say, 'Oh, I shouldn't be feeling that' and you don't go into denial about it. In inquiry, we are happy simply to find out what is *actually* going on.

As you do this inquiry, relax into your experience. Allow yourself to *be with* whatever you are experiencing without thinking too much about it. This is how your awareness is showing up in this moment.

The tool of investigation is the question, and a powerful tool it is. In every kind of work, in every walk of life, asking the right question is the key.

We ask, 'What is under the surface here, under the appearance?' There is always a deeper level. Having a murky conversation with someone, you might ask yourself, 'What is this person *really* saying?' and suddenly gain clarity. You might ask yourself, 'What does this person want?' Or more importantly, 'What do *I* want?'—to become aware of your true intentionality. Fundamentally, every one of us has, in our deepest nature, the desire to know who we are, the desire to know the Self. And even when we want some kind of external gratification, we are really looking for the peace and bliss of the Self. We want money, we want to feel secure. What is feeling secure? It is an attribute of the Self. We want love, we want to feel love. Whose love do you feel? You feel your own love, actually. You want that awakening of love within. All these are attributes of the Self: the love, the peace, the wisdom, the light, the acceptance and the contentment are all within us, and that is what we seek. Along with the question, 'What's going on here?' remember to make use of the question, 'Who is in here?' Has another person crept into your inner space?

RECOGNITION

After investigation, there is recognition. Recognition is the simple acknowledgment of what *is*. It is an experimental attitude. In investigation, we asked the question, 'What is going on?' Now we answer it. The tool of recognition is my beloved A-Statement. The A-Statement is much misunderstood. Everyone wants to leap to God with no groundwork. They want to transcend without dealing with material reality. If only it were possible! There is an old blues song that goes, 'Everybody wants to get to heaven but nobody wants to die'.

You cannot get to heaven unless you make the proper A-Statements. G-Statements like 'I am the Self. I am Brahman. I am God' lack punch if you have not yet first located yourself in truth, in the most mundane way. The A-Statement is a reality check. It says, 'I feel mad, sad, bad, scared or glad'. It bears witness to where you are; it locates you in present time.

Patanjali describes one type of delusion, called *viparyaya*, the delusion borne of words. When I first read that in Patanjali, I felt I had wasted 20 years in *viparyaya*. I had been intoxicated by intellectual constructions, believing I was attaining the truth that way. Ungrounded thought and ungrounded language carry you away from the Self because they take you out of the present moment. On the other hand, feelings and sensations, attention to the breath, and awareness of the senses bring you present.

I am not denigrating the intellect and the mind because when they are used properly, they are a powerful means of knowing the Self. But they can also be delusive. They can take you right away from the truth and the Self. The A-Statement always grounds you in present reality.

There is an A-Statement sutra in *Spanda Karikas*:

> *Aham sukhi cha duhkhi cha raktashcha ityadisamvidaha*
> *sukhadyavasthanusyute vartante 'nyatra taha sphutam.*

> I am happy, I am miserable, I am attached—these and other cognitions have their being evidently in another in which the states of happiness, misery etc. are strung together.

'I am happy, I am miserable, I am attached'. These are clearly A-Statements. The sutra says that there is a Self that underlies the different mental and emotional moods. These states must come from somewhere and not thin air. That somewhere is the Self or Consciousness.

Underneath each A-Statement like 'I am happy' or 'I am miserable' is the Self. The different states can be seen as waves on the ocean of Self. When you see islands in the sea, you know they don't come up from nothing, they point to a land mass that joins them under the sea.

Common to A-Statements like 'I am angry. I am sad. I am scared', in fact, to all A-Statements, is the statement 'I am', which we explored in Lecture 2. You could say that 'I am' is the supreme A-Statement. Some yogis contemplate the 'I am' and try not to descend into the emotions. While this method is heroic, it tends not to deal with life issues, which are critical to everyone, even great yogis. At the level of the 'I am', the A-Statement merges with the G-Statement: 'I am' is the supreme non-reducible A-Statement and also a profound G-Statement.

The sutra says it's okay to feel 'I am happy', it's okay to feel 'I am sad', it's okay to feel 'I am angry' because these are simply permutations of the original truth. If used rightly, these words and these states can lead back to the original truth. If they are an outgrowth or a transformation, they can bring you to the Self. They can provide a trail back. You say, 'I know who you really are, Mr Depression. You are really the Self, if I know how to follow you. I am going to follow you and see what you do in the woods. There you are in your dark little hut being depressed, being miserable. And then late at night, something else happens and you become blissful. Yes, I'm following you!'

In this second part of Self-inquiry, recognition, you locate the feeling. Go inside and feel what is there. What is the feeling? I like to objectify it—make it an object and really experience it like a thing. Sometimes when I do private work (which is a form of 'interior coaching'), I ask a person, 'What does it feel like? What size is it?' Because I'm a boy, I say, 'Is it like a cricket ball or a basketball? What shape is it? What colour is it? What is it made of?' in order to give it a concrete form. For an expanded version of a Shiva Process Self-inquiry private session, see Appendix I.

The next important step is to understand that this feeling is actually made of *matrika*. It is made of emotions, and it has a story in it, and attitudes. Your depression is like that, or your anger. It's got a whole story and a whole collection of intellectual and emotional content. If it is a negative feeling, it also has wrong understanding in it. Why? Because if it had the right understanding, you would feel bliss and peace.

If I get something like that inside myself, I love it. I say, 'Happy day!' I have something to inquire into. What joy! I ask it questions and I let it speak to me, always knowing that underneath it is the Self. That is how inquiry arose within me in my relationship with my Guru. So, calmly look for what is there, knowing full well that the Self lies under it. There is nothing to fear.

That was a pristine bit of one-minute inquiry. This is recognition. You see how simple and direct inquiry is? Just looking and seeing. Even if you don't feel as though you understand the technical aspects of it, just do it. Look within and observe.

One more thing, before we move on. Last night after the talk, someone in the audience told me that he'd done quite a bit of Neuro-linguistic programming, and he's a visual type of person. Accordingly, it's hard for him to get in touch with feeling in the centres; instead, he gets images. I agree with NLP that there are some who are more oriented to the visual, others to feeling, and then there are those who lean towards the tactile or kinesthetic. Any of these modes can work for inquiry. I dug up an interesting report that one of our facilitators sent me on just such a private session.

The facilitator wrote:

> The player expressed the emotions in her throat, a constricted area for her, as looking like a bag of Liquorice

Allsorts. I asked what these lollies represented. She replied that they were made of different sorts of feelings, thoughts and experiences. I asked if she had taken a bite out of any of them and she answered: 'Some are whole, but some I have partially eaten. I like this kind of lolly, so they aren't bad, but I would rather digest them all. They seem uncomfortably stuck in this area.'

We then moved to the 'lolly' that' seemed the most urgent, and the player reported that it represented feelings about her family. We used A- and B-Statements and then I asked her to repicture the space in the throat chakra. She described it as a 'free-flowing sweet black stream of liquorice', saying, 'all the lollies are now one and are streaming towards my heart'.

That's an interesting account from several points of view. I'm highlighting it because the facilitator was clever enough to move with the player's predilection for the visual over the emotional.

UPLIFTMENT AND TRANSFORMATION

The third stage of inquiry is upliftment and transformation; 'upliftment' involves spiritual transformation. This is the arena of the faculty of imagination. Now we move closer to the goal: we want to have an upward shift—*unmesha*—and we want to go deeper. We want to find the underlying spiritual truth. We want the limitations of ego to dissolve into the joy of the Self. We want the feeling of contraction and disempowerment to become empowerment and expansion.

The tool of upliftment and transformation is the B-, G- and D-Statement. These are the statements that uplift. As we have outlined, an A-Statement locates where you are, while a B-, G- or D-Statement takes you further. A conventional B-Statement reassures you or makes you feel better about yourself, while G-Statements come from high spiritual sources. Scripture gives G-Statements like *Aham Brahmasmi*: 'I am the Absolute.' And we shouldn't forget the D-Statement, which uplifts by telling us what needs to be done, and transforms through action.

The first job of a person who is doing inquiry, if they are in a negative space, is to return to peace. The more committed you are to inquiry, the more you will make that your priority. Let's investigate the upward shift.

**TRACK 13. INQUIRY:
LOOKING FOR THE UPWARD SHIFT INSIDE**

Close your eyes and search for feelings or ideas within yourself. Is there joy inside (confidence, satisfaction, pleasure)? Is there love inside (gratitude)? Is there clarity or wisdom inside? Is there peace or contentment inside? Is there energy inside? Is there doership or ambition inside? In each case, locate where in the body the feeling is held.

If you are a seasoned meditator, you have probably experienced the state of *nirvikalpa samadhi*. *Nirvikalpa* means the *samadhi* with 'no *vikalpas*', no thought-forms. This same state is sometimes called *nirbija samadhi*; that is, the *samadhi* without 'seed' (*bija*). The seed referred to is, again, thought-forms. There is a *samadhi* beyond even these two. It is a *samadhi* in which the eyes remain open and thought-forms may still play in the mind. It is called *sahaja samadhi*. Beings absorbed in *sahaja samadhi* have attained the goal of spirituality. Even though they may have to deal with all the diverse challenges of their mundane life, they remain at peace and centred in the Self. They do not experience depletion or depression, but only the expansion of love.

To experience the *sahaja* state is to live an awakened life. When you do that, there is tremendous energy. You are present in your life, not lost in a dream. In sport it is called 'the zone'. Athletes train their whole lives to spend 10 minutes in the zone where everything clicks. Their consciousness is poised, their body responsive and relaxed; everything works. They don't know how they got there. All too soon, they lose it and they don't know how they lost it. Martial arts, of course, is based on that. Martial artists train their mind and body so they can 'do without doing'; so they can enter a mind-free state and flow with what comes up. Indeed, this word 'flow' conveys a sense of the *sahaja* state.

When true inquiry awakens and *sahaja samadhi* is attained, we become like the poet-saint Kabir who says:

> Oh *sadhus*, oh seekers, wherever I see, I see God alone. Wherever I walk, I walk around God. Whatever I do is an act of worship to Him.

Kabir is saying, I live with oneness, I don't live at war with my environment. I don't see threat, I don't see paranoia everywhere. I am at home. For example, when you are by yourself in your own living room, you feel at ease. At least I hope you feel at ease there. So, the whole universe is my living room. I am so much at ease in my own skin. I am at ease with myself. If you do spiritual practice, you add something to what *is*. But if you are in the natural state, everything is already 'it'. There is nowhere to go, nothing to do. There is no place to be; you are already there.

When our contemplation is perfect, when our inquiry is profound, we reach that natural state. We attain that joy and that flow. How do we do it? Through inquiry, through contemplation, through awareness, through focus; this is the secret.

You know that if you act out of negativity, it will have negative effects. If you are angry and you interact with people, you will communicate anger and create negative effects. As the seed, so the fruit. This is true of all actions that flow from negative emotions.

Intelligent people make peace their first priority. When they attain peace, their minds are more reliable. When they are under the sway of anger or fear, their minds are untrustworthy. Paranoia deludes us. It makes us see things that aren't there. You might have had the experience of believing that some person hates you and gossips about you, and then you find out that it was completely untrue. Have you ever had that experience? Or have you found out that it *is* true? That's not paranoia, that's insight! But, even then, you should have right understanding and know that it is not really you. That person is really talking to somebody seven lifetimes ago. You are just standing in for them—you're the proxy.

When you are in a state of peace, you have an understanding based in peace—live it with conviction. Go right forward. You need not worry or hold back: if those intuitions turn out to be false, you'll know it. They will pull you away from peace. You will know what you have to do.

IMAGINATION

The arena of spiritual upliftment is that of grace, and it is also the realm of the creative use of the imagination. In our culture, the imaginative faculty and artists who possess it to a high degree are much admired. There is good reason for this. People you know who are entirely lacking imagination live in a narrow and deadened universe. People with powerful imaginations live in a world full of energy and possibility. But imagination can go off the rails. When coloured by fear, it becomes paranoia or hypochondria. When vitiated by ego, it becomes inflated and delusional. Even in the case of creative artists, imagination is trivialised when it is undisciplined and self-indulgent; that is, when it is not connected to the practical realities of life.

Of all the uses of imagination, the most noble is the yogi's use of the G- Statement. It is precisely the imaginative faculty, the faculty of intuition, that the yogi uses to connect with a higher reality. Thus, the yogi is the supreme performance artist whose supreme work of art is the inner Self. Self-realisation contains all the emotions of great art: the joy of comedy, the love of romance, the splendour of epic and the power of adventure.

The Shaivite knows that G-Statements like 'I am the Self. I am Shiva. I am Consciousness' point to the fundamental truth. That is all one needs to contemplate. When my teacher told me to say, 'I am the Self. I am Shiva', that became my creative contemplation for many years, and even to this day.

If we find ourselves in a negative space, our first job as practitioners of inquiry is to return to peace, straight away. The more deeply committed we are to inquiry, the more we will make that our priority. When we use B- and G- Statements, we affirm the power of imagination, the power of the spirit, and use it to overcome doubt, just as artists must overcome obstacles to bring their vision to fruition.

Making a G- Statement implies an inner yoga. I say inwardly, 'I am Shiva'. A voice responds, 'No! You are not' or 'How can that be?' Moving at the speed of light, the imagination works on behalf of the G- Statement, finding ways to justify the higher truth that 'You are Shiva' and empower it. The great beings bear witness to that truth, and the battle is won in your inner world by earnestness and practice.

TABLE: STAGES OF SELF-INQUIRY

These, then, are the three stages of Self-inquiry: investigation, recognition, and upliftment and transformation. They are associated with the question (investigation), the A-Statement (recognition) and the B-, G- and D-Statement (upliftment and transformation).

I have put these in a table for easier reference:

Stage I	Stage II	Stage III
INVESTIGATION	**RECOGNITION**	**UPLIFTMENT & TRANSFORMATION**
Includes: Observation & Inquiry	Includes: Testing/Experimenting & Acknowledgment	Includes: Imagination & Action
Technique used: Looking & Questioning	Technique used: A-Statement	Technique used: B-, G- & D-Statements

In investigation, the task is to answer the question 'What's going on here?' In short, to look at what *is*. In recognition, the task is to determine the nature of what *is* in a most basic and practical way in terms of feeling: I feel this. I feel that. Upliftment and transformation use the basic reality uncovered in recognition as a jumping-off point. They affirm that behind the basic reality of the A-Statement is a deeper and always present spiritual truth; a higher reality hidden beneath the surface reality. Finally, we touch that deeper reality. This stage we call upliftment and transformation, but it could as easily be called resolution or grace. For a breakdown of the key questions of Self-inquiry, see Appendix H.

THE POWER OF LANGUAGE: 'FEEDING THE RIGHT DOG'

Behind all of inquiry is the indispensable insight that we create our own reality by the use of language, both inwardly and outwardly. *Spanda Karikas* says:

> *Shabdarashi-samutthasya shaktivargasya bhogyatam*
> *Kalavilupta-vibhavo gataha san sa pashuhu smrtah.*

> Being deprived of his glory by *kalaa*, he (the individual) becomes a victim of the group of powers arising from the multitude of words, and thus he is known as the bound one.

The aphorism says we are deprived of our glory, our Shiva nature, by a group of malevolent letters and words inside our brain, which diminish and imprison us. What a fabulous conception! I envision these letters like an animated cartoon character or Darth Vader as *matrika*.

Another sutra says:

> *Svarupavarane chasya shaktayaha satatotthitaha*
> *Yataha shabdanuvedhena na vina pratyayodbhavaha.*

> *Brahmi* and other powers are ever in readiness to conceal [a person's] real nature, for without the association of words, ideas cannot arise.

'*Brahmi* and other powers' are the powers of the alphabet, of language. It is as though language is crouching within you in subtle form, ready for the opportunity to delude you. Isn't that frightening? Marvellous stuff for the ninth century!

As *Spanda Karikas* says:

> *Seyam kriyatmika shaktihi shivasya pashuvartini*
> *Bandhayitri svamargastha jnata siddhyupapadika.*

> That aforementioned operative power of Shiva existing in the bound soul is a source of bondage; the same when realised as residing in him as the way of approach to one's own essential reality brings about success (i.e. the achievement of liberation).

That very same language power, when we understand it correctly and use it properly, can bring us to liberation. We don't have to hate our minds or become alienated from our thought-making ability. If we use it properly, it can uplift us.

Language is bondage, but it is also a means to liberation. Through the mind, bondage; through the mind, liberation. The mind is a double-bladed axe: it has its good side and its bad side. It is dualistic. The dark and light are both within us.

In a detective novel I read, a character named Harry Bosch says that we have two dogs inside of us, a good dog and a bad dog. One dog goes towards the light and one dog goes to the dark side.

When we indulge our tearing thoughts and hence our depression, we are 'feeding the wrong dog'. When we remember the teachings and the Self, we are 'feeding the right dog'. The choice is ultimately our own.

Perhaps there is a person you hate; a person who gives you negative feedback all the time. Then you have a breakthrough and change your attitude and your behaviour, and maybe apologise or do whatever is necessary, and suddenly the person becomes full of love. Now you're feeding the right dog. Have you had that experience? Deities are like that. If you propitiate them, they open doors for you, but if you don't have their grace, look out! Lord Ganesh is said to remove obstacles, but few know that under certain circumstances, He creates obstacles.

The letters of the alphabet are like that. Sometimes they are mean and nasty and they give you tearing thoughts—but if you treat them right, they give you uplifting thoughts; they give you G-Statements; they give you self-esteem. You have to treat them right. You have to educate them. You have to speak sweetly to them.

Self-hatred is public enemy number one in spiritual life. Remember that Shiva is within you, and don't dishonour supreme Consciousness by lack of self-acceptance. If you love others, but you hate yourself, then think of yourself as *other*. You see, to other people you are an 'other'. Be as nice to your mind as you are to an 'other' whom you love. Say, 'Oh my mind, think positive thoughts. Oh my mind, think positive thoughts'.

TRACK 14.
CONTEMPLATION: SPEAKING TO YOUR MIND

Say to yourself:

- Oh my mind, think positive thoughts.

- Think well of me.

- Think well of others.

Notice the feeling tone that comes with each of these three statements.

The text we have been looking at, the *Spanda Karikas*, says there are forces of delusion within our universe. These forces exist outwardly, but they also exist inwardly within our own Consciousness. They manifest themselves through the negative power of language. At the same time, the *Spanda Karikas* gives hints as to how to fight against these forces. The following sutra lies at the heart of Shaivite yoga, personal inquiry and group-inquiry. It says:

> *Ataha satatam udyuktaha spanda-tattva-viviktaye*
> *Jagradeva nijam bhavam achirenadhigachchati*
>
> Therefore, one should be always on the alert for the discernment of the *spanda* principle. Such a person attains his essential state (as *spanda*) even in the waking condition in short time.

The *spanda* principle is the principle of the expansion of Consciousness. Most fundamentally, it refers to the actual vibration of enlightenment, joy and illumination that occurs when a meditator connects with the Self. Regarded more generally, every positive movement in the universe, mundane as well as spiritual, is part of the *spanda* principle.

Every success we have, every time things go well, every little joy or pleasure, has a bit of *spanda* and that is why we value them. But most of these positive movements are based on temporary things, and they are fleeting or mixed with negative factors. The purest and most pristine form of the *spanda* principle is the expansion of awareness and the upliftment of the heart that comes from mystic union, a deep inner connectedness.

Practitioners of personal inquiry must carefully watch their inner world and its contractions and expansions. In the same way, participants in group-inquiry watch the movement of Consciousness within the room, always seeking the *spanda* principle.

Finally, *Spanda Karikas* says:

> *Tada tasmin mahavyomni pralinashashibhaskare*
> *Saushupta-padavan mudhah prabuddhah syadanavrtah*

> Taking firm hold of that (*spanda*) the awakened yogi remains firm with the resolution, 'I will surely carry out whatever it will tell me'.

The yogis of inquiry commit themselves to live and die by the *spanda* principle; the upward shift of feeling, the expansion of Consciousness. In so doing, they separate from the mass of humanity living superficially in externals and egoic self-interest. The *spanda* principle is the watermark of the Divine discerned within. Following it constitutes devotion to the expansion of divine Consciousness, and raises a practitioner to a higher level of being. You no longer evaluate life according to external success or failure, but by the pulsation of *spanda*, the quality of aliveness.

Resolutely attending to this practice, seekers build wisdom power. They have not only intellectual understanding of the inner path but they become effective in practical life as well. Their emotions become serene and uplifted. They purify their faculties of will/emotion, understanding and action. They live happily in touch with the inner principle and become empowered in all areas of life.

This is the real worship of the Self. Pay attention to your inner process. In ritual worship, various materials like ghee, incense and a light are offered to the deity. But the highest worship is to offer attention. Wherever we put our attention, whatever we take interest in, is our God. If our interest is money, and we brood about money, then Mammon is our God. If we take interest in our inner life, and work in our inner world, then we are yogis.

See God in others. In relating to others, strengthen kindness with truth, humanise truth with kindness.

Yogis of Self-inquiry are present to life. They are a fire. They say:

> Throw out *religion*, which belongs to the dead, dusty past and seek *revelation*.
>
> Throw out *philosophy*, which belongs to the slow, stupid mind and seek *insight*.
>
> Throw out *nostalgia* and *sentimentality*, and find *love*.
>
> The wisdom voice that speaks in scriptures and through the sages is also in you.
>
> That great experience you once had is available now as well.
>
> The world you want to transform stands already transformed.
>
> The person you want to become is already you.
>
> There is no person, no thought, no object and no emotion that is not Shiva.

Everything rests and has its being in supreme Consciousness. When you know this viscerally, you are free. Don't settle for the periphery of life. Be more profound. Meditate, contemplate, investigate—go deeper. Inquire into your present experience until the delight of the inner Self floods your heart.

SUMMARY

- Yoga is about connecting with the inner power.

- Ignorance causes depression.

- The Self is always present.

- Self-inquiry is about awareness.

- There are three movements to inquiry: investigation; recognition; upliftment and transformation.

- Investigation involves observation (looking) and inquiry (questioning).

- The tool of investigation is the question.

- Recognition involves testing and experimenting.

- Recognition is the acknowledgment of what *is* by means of the A-Statement.

- Upliftment and transformation use the faculty of imagination.

- The tool of upliftment and transformation is the B-, G- and D-Statement.

- We create our experience through our inner language.

- Feed the right dog.

- The *spanda* principle is the watermark of the Divine discerned within.

- In Self-inquiry, we watch inner contractions and expansions.

- There is nothing that is not Shiva or Consciousness.

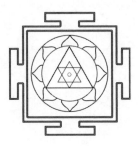

AFTERWORD

I'VE SPOKEN A lot about Self-inquiry in both its individual and group forms. Reading this book, you could easily get the idea that it's a technical and complicated matter. Now, at the end, I'd like to affirm that this is not the case at all. Inquiry is simple and direct. You begin where you are in the present moment with whatever thoughts and feelings you discover when you turn within. Systematically, by means of questions and insight, you unpack those thoughts and feelings, and hear the messages they give you. Doing this, the tension generated by fear and frustration is relaxed. That which is hidden underneath, in all its joy and *spanda*, is revealed. My friends, pay attention to what is inside you. Go deeper. Look for that which is most inclusive and noble. The truth is harmonious. Discover it.

A-STATEMENTS

BASIC A-STATEMENTS ARE:

- I feel mad, sad, bad, scared or glad.

FURTHER A-STATEMENTS INCLUDE:

- I feel furious.
- I feel content.
- I feel loving.
- I feel calm.
- I feel illumined.
- I feel jealous.
- I feel bored.
- I feel fascinated.
- I feel disgusted.
- I feel worried.

B-STATEMENTS

- I am worthy.
- I am a good person.
- I'm nice looking.
- My mother loves me.
- 'I'm OK-You're OK.'
- I give my best.
- I'll get over it.
- I forgive myself.
- I accept myself.
- I've got a lot to offer.

G-STATEMENTS

- Everything is Consciousness.
- Consciousness is the dearest, most healing and desirable thing.
- I am Shiva.
- Every thought and feeling, even my blocks, are Shiva.
- Wherever the mind goes is Shiva.
- The whole world is inside my own awareness.
- My thought-forms create my experience of life.
- I am the Lord of Matrika.
- I am the Lord of my own *shaktis*.
- This universe is Shiva's grace.
- This universe is drenched in love.
- There is no distinction between worldly and spiritual.
- There is absolutely no problem.
- There is nothing outside of Consciousness.
- I am Shiva and my mind, senses and emotions are *shaktis*.
- Every other person is Shiva, too.
- The form of Consciousness never changes.
- All these people are Shiva in their universe.
- There is no obstruction to Shiva anywhere.
- Nothing veils Shiva—He is apparent.
- All my feelings are permutations of bliss.
- Whatever gives me peace or satisfaction shows me Shiva.
- My mind does not exist.

- I am everywhere.

- There is no bondage and no liberation.

- Everything is perfect as it is.

- Shiva's grace is the only thing I need.

- Everything is going according to Shiva's plan.

- The present state is Shiva in that form.

- Whatever meditation I am having is Shiva.

- The object is contained within the subject.

- No outer event can harm my true nature.

- Shiva is my most intimate inner space.

- O Shiva, give me your grace!

- O Shakti, O Mother, be kind to me!

- I open my heart completely to the experience of Shiva.

- Right now, exactly as I am, I am Shiva.

APPENDIX D (TRACK 15—read by Ma Devi)

SELF-INQUIRY
FOR THE FOUR AREAS OF LIFE

THE AREAS OF LIFE CAN BE DIVIDED INTO:

1. **Health/Body**

2. **Career**

3. **Relationship/Family**

4. **Spirituality (which underlies all of them).**

1. HEALTH/BODY

- Bring your body into your awareness.

- Make the statement, 'I give myself permission to hear the answers of the Self'.

- Divide the body into sections: the head and throat, the chest, the stomach, the genital region, the legs and feet, and the arms.

- Close your eyes and locate any feeling of physical disease or discomfort in the body.

- Make an A-Statement: 'I feel sickness/pain in my head. I feel sickness/pain in my stomach.'

- What do I need to do about this?
    - Do I need to see a doctor or a practitioner?
    - Do I need to take medicine or a remedy?
    - Do I need to change my diet?
    - Is the condition psychological?
    - What is one step I can take to feel healthier?
        - Should I walk more?
        - Should I do yoga?

- Should I swim?
- Should I jog?
- Which exercise might give me more energy?
- Do I need to change my diet?
- Do I need to be more disciplined in my diet?
- What food should I stay away from?
- What food should I embrace?
- How can I accept and love my body more?

2. CAREER

- Bring your work, service or career into your awareness.

- Make the statement, 'I give myself permission to hear the answers of the Self'.

- Where inside you does the block in your career seem to show up?

  - Is this block sadness, fear or anger?

  - Make an A-Statement.

  - Do I need to communicate something to someone?

  - Do I need to forgive someone at work?

  - Do I need to change my attitude?

  - Do I need advice or help in this area?

  - Do I need to take a break?

  - What is one step I can take to increase my creativity or interest at work?

  - Do I need to change jobs?

  - Does the block have to do with money?

    - Do I need to spend less?

    - Do I need to spend more?

3. RELATIONSHIP/FAMILY

- Bring your relationships into your awareness.

- Make the statement, 'I give myself permission to hear the answers of the Self'.

- Where inside you does the block in your relationships seem to show up?

  - Do I need to forgive myself or someone else?

  - Is there a conversation I need to have?

  - Make an A-Statement.

  - Am I carrying some of that person's pain?

  - Do I need to change my attitude?

  - Do I need to give something up?

  - Do I need to accept something?

  - Do I need to give more love?

  - Do I need to spend more time with that person?

  - Do I need to love that person in my meditation?

4. SPIRITUALITY

- Bring your spiritual life into your awareness.

- Make the statement, 'I give myself permission to hear the answers of the Self'.

- Am I growing spiritually or am I blocked?

- Where in my body does the block show up?

- How can I get rid of the block and increase the Shakti?

  - Do I need to meditate more?

  - Do I need to be more authentic?

  - Do I need to let something go?

  - Do I need to accept something?

APPENDIX E (TRACK 1)

SELF-INQUIRY
GUIDED CHAKRA MEDITATION

I suggest that you try and listen to this meditation and the following healing meditation every day during the time you read this book. Set aside at least 20 minutes daily. This will assist your practice and help develop Self-inquiry naturally.

1. NAVEL CHAKRA

■ Bring your attention to the navel chakra. Feel the feeling in the navel area.

- ◆ Is it pleasant or unpleasant?
- ◆ Is it tense or relaxed?
- ◆ Is it calm or energised?
- ◆ Is there a feeling of wanting or pushing?
- ◆ Is there a feeling of harmony or struggle?
- ◆ Be aware of the feelings in the navel area.

2. HEART CHAKRA

■ Bring your attention to the heart chakra. Feel the feeling in the heart chakra.

- ◆ Is it pleasant or unpleasant?
- ◆ Is it sad or happy or some other feeling?
- ◆ Is the heart open or closed?
- ◆ Is it loving or withholding?
- ◆ Feel the feelings in the heart chakra.

3. THROAT CHAKRA

■ Bring your attention to the throat chakra. Feel the feeling in the throat.

- Is it pleasant or unpleasant?
- Is it blocked or open?
- Are words or emotion caught there?
- Feel the feelings in the throat chakra.

4. THIRD-EYE CHAKRA

■ Bring your attention to the third eye, the point between the eyebrows.

- Is it pleasant or unpleasant?
- Is it tense or relaxed?
- Is there confusion or worry?
- Is it expanded or contracted?
- Is it light or dark?
- Do you see any colours?
- Feel the feelings in the third-eye chakra.

Review the four chakras you have just surveyed and determine which of them is the best or most comfortable and which is the worst or least comfortable.

APPENDIX F (TRACK 2)

HEALING MEDITATION

1. NAVEL CHAKRA

- Get in touch with the feeling in the navel chakra. The navel has to do with issues of will. Sometimes it becomes tense when we are resisting divine will.

    - Relax the navel and say, 'I let go. I relax. I surrender'.

    - Imagine yourself floating on a calm lake.

    - Let the current gently take you and say, 'Everything will be okay'.

    - Bring in the thought 'I feel safe and relaxed'.

2. HEART CHAKRA

- Now feel the feeling in the heart chakra. The proper function of the heart chakra is to love. Contemplate love and forgiveness.

    - Bring in the thought 'I let my heart open' or 'I call on the power of love'.

    - Practise forgiving and accepting yourself. Bring in the thoughts 'I forgive myself. I accept myself'.

    - Let go of grievances against people who have hurt you. You can say, 'I am willing to forgive those who have hurt me'.

    - Ask for forgiveness from those whom you may have hurt consciously or unconsciously. You can say, 'Please forgive me, I forgive you'.

    - Let love expand and say inwardly, 'I give my love'.

3. THROAT CHAKRA

- Bring your attention to the throat chakra. The throat chakra has to do with communication of words and feelings. Say to yourself the following statements:

- I communicate my thoughts and feelings.

- I say what I need to say to the people whom I need to.

- I speak with truth and kindness.

- I speak powerful and loving words.

4. THIRD-EYE CHAKRA

■ Bring your awareness to the third eye. Become aware of the feeling in the third eye. The third eye is the centre of wisdom and insight. Say to yourself:

- I open my mind to higher wisdom.

- I open to truth.

- My mind is illumined.

- Wisdom is within me.

- I see the truth.

To conclude the meditation, you can select the most positive chakra and contemplate it for the rest of your meditation period. You can play some gentle meditative music or sacred chanting as a background for your practice.

OPENING STATEMENTS AND CLOSING QUESTIONS IN GROUP-INQUIRY

BEFORE THE GROUP:

- I dedicate myself to speaking the truth.

- I dedicate myself to speaking the truth with kindness.

- I dedicate myself to helping others know the true Self.

- I dedicate myself to knowing the true Self.

- I rededicate myself to the essence of *sadhana*.

- I honour everything that arises as the play of Consciousness.

- I carefully watch the movement of Shakti within and without.

- I seek the highest wisdom in each situation.

AT THE END OF THE GROUP:

- Are you carrying anything?

- Did you see more than you said?

- Do you want to praise anyone?

- Do you want to blame anyone?

- Are you worried about anyone?

- Did you want to say anything to anyone?

- Were you able to say what you needed to say?

- Was there truth?

- Was there falsity?

- Do you want to apologise to anyone?

- Did anger, fear or sadness arise in you or in the group?

- Did the group touch a mystery?

- Did you see God or evidence of God?

- Was there equal measure of truth and kindness?

- Were you present: All? A lot? Some? Little?

- Did the feeling move up? Did the feeling move down?

- What was the high point of the group in feeling and interest?

- Do you have advice for anyone?

- Did you have a yogic or practical understanding?

- Do you or does anyone need homework?

SIX KEY QUESTIONS OF SELF-INQUIRY

The Shiva Process method of Self-inquiry can be neatly and swiftly summarised as a series of six questions.

THE SIX QUESTIONS ARE:

1. What's going on here? (Investigation)

2. What emotion is it? (Recognition; A-Statement)

3. What caused it? (Story)

4. What do I need to do to change the feeling, to relax the contraction? (Story; four things to do in a bad situation)

5. What understanding do I need to release the contraction? (Resolution; B-Statement/D-Statement)

6. What is the highest perspective I can take? (Upliftment and Transformation; G-Statement)

1. WHAT'S GOING ON HERE? (INVESTIGATION)

With this question, you focus on contracted feeling within. You may have to overcome your resistance to do this.

- Which chakra is the feeling in?
  - navel?
  - heart?
  - throat?
  - third eye?

- Describe it closely:
  - size
  - shape
  - colour
  - material

In this stage, you isolate and locate a contracted feeling and observe it closely. Get as close to it as possible.

2. WHAT EMOTION IS IT? (RECOGNITION; A-STATEMENT)

Because it is a contracted feeling, it is a negative emotion and it is usually a form of anger, fear or sorrow. For example, self-hatred is anger turned within; jealousy is a form of anger which contains self-hatred that comes about when someone else gets what you want. Yogically considered, all negative emotions are some subvariant of the original polarity of attachment and aversion.

- Make your A-Statement.

3. WHAT CAUSED IT? (STORY)

- What interface with the world caused this emotion?
- Was it something in the past, present or future?
- Was it an event that happened today or recently?
- Is it a chronic situation?
- A job issue?
- A relationship issue?
- A body issue?
- A spiritual issue?
- You've now located the story element.

4. WHAT DO I NEED TO DO TO CHANGE THE FEELING, TO RELAX THE CONTRACTION? (STORY; FOUR THINGS TO DO IN A BAD SITUATION)

- Change the situation (speak up, have a new plan and so on).
- Leave the situation (not always possible but sometimes necessary).
- Change your attitude (surrender to something, accept something, get off something, and so on).

- Do nothing. (Everything is shifting and changing. Finally, at some point, an alignment happens. While the elevator is going up or down, you can do nothing but wait. Eventually, the elevator reaches the right floor, a door opens and you can walk through.)

5. WHAT UNDERSTANDING DO I NEED TO RELEASE THE CONTRACTION? (RESOLUTION; B- AND D-STATEMENT)

- If there's something that you see you can do in the external situation, resolve now to do it: 'I resolve to speak with Peter.' This homework is your D-Statement (remember that a D-Statement, an action statement, is a form of B-Statement that commits you to a specific action).

- Similarly, if leaving a situation is what you need to do, that becomes your D-Statement: 'I resolve to leave.'

- If an inner change is necessary, allow your intuition to find a B-Statement that works:

  - I accept him.

  - I forgive her.

  - I will not beat on closed doors.

  - I am content with what I have.

  - I will not pursue rejection.

  - I accept the reality.

  - I let go of the past.

  - I trust in the future.

  - Everything is okay.

6. WHAT IS THE HIGHEST PERSPECTIVE I CAN TAKE? (UPLIFTMENT AND TRANSFORMATION; G-STATEMENT)

- Find a transpersonal spiritual statement that takes you beyond your personal desire and fear, likes and dislikes:

- I surrender to God.
- Jesus loves me.
- All this will pass.
- Everything is the play of Consciousness.
- It's all an illusion.
- I call on the Self.
- God, please help me.

A SHIVA PROCESS SELF-INQUIRY PRIVATE SESSION

Every individual session of Shiva Process is different, since it is an engagement with the play of Consciousness. The following outlines a potent technique that has evolved over many years, but need not be followed slavishly.

1. OPENING CHAT

At the beginning of the session, the facilitator chats with the player, trying to establish the area of inquiry. Is this a general session or does the player want to focus on a specific area of life (for example, health, career, relationship) or a specific issue within one of those areas? Narrowing the field of inquiry is helpful, but a general spiritual inquiry is also effective. Sometimes, during inquiry, deeper issues are discovered which the player was not conscious of.

2. GUIDED INQUIRY

If a specific area of life has been determined, the facilitator asks the player to contemplate that area in a general way. If a particular issue has been determined, again, the facilitator asks the player to contemplate that issue. Now, the facilitator leads the player through an investigation of the feeling in the navel, heart, throat and third-eye chakras. The player's eyes are closed during this time to focus attention on the inner world. Is each of these centres tense or relaxed? Is the feeling pleasant or unpleasant? The player answers the question silently.

3. RESULTS OF INQUIRY

Now, with the eyes open, the player is asked which chakra was the most tense or unpleasant. This becomes the focus of the next stage.

4. INVESTIGATING THE BLOCK

Both the player and facilitator close their eyes. The player now answers the facilitator's questions out loud.

The player should focus on the worst chakra. Through the next series of questions, the facilitator brings the player as close as possible to the block.

- How large is the block?

- If it were made of a physical substance, what would it be made of? (Choose from whatever springs to mind: wood, rubber, metal, water, feathers and so on.)

- Does it have a colour?

- What emotion is it? (Since it's a contracted feeling, the emotion will be some permutation of anger, fear, sadness or disgust.)

- What caused it? (It could be a recent event or a chronic situation.)

5. FEEDBACK: FINDING THE A-STATEMENTS

Now the player is ready to make A-Statements given by the facilitator. These can be pure statements of present feeling ('I feel angry' or 'I feel sad') or hybrid statements that include elements of the story ('I'm angry at my boss' or 'My wife hurt my feelings').

It is important for the facilitator to remember that the Shiva Process is not an advice-giving session and they should serve the actual feeling of the player, and not the facilitator's thoughts or feelings about that feeling. Sometimes a shift can happen by strange and unique means and not by rational or linear methods.

6. WIDENING THE DISCUSSION

Finding the A-Statements allows the player to delve deeper into their issues and, at appropriate moments, more feedback, in the form of A-statements, can be given.

7. B-STATEMENTS

When the facilitator senses that the essential issues have been discovered and expressed, they can move to B-Statements, seeking a solution or upward shift. These can be feeling statements ('I'm good at what I do' or 'I love my wife') or D-Statements that involve homework assignments ('I will have a meeting with X' or 'I will tell my wife I love her').

8. CONCLUSION

Having unblocked the flow of feeling and expression, a relaxed and comprehensive culminating discussion will follow. In some cases, a number of these steps may have to be repeated as deeper layers of truth are revealed, and surprising and unexpected elements come into play. In fact, this is one of the pleasures of inquiry: things are often not what they seem, and hidden causes may be operating. Remember, however, to recognise and be satisfied with a shift.

APPENDIX J (CD TRACK LISTING)

SUMMARY OF RECORDED INQUIRIES AND CONTEMPLATIONS

Track 1. Appendix E: Self-Inquiry Guided Chakra Meditation

Track 2. Appendix F: Healing Meditation

Track 3. Inquiry: Reviewing Your Day

Track 4. Inquiry: Who Am I?

Track 5. Contemplation: Becoming Present

Track 6. Contemplation: You Can Always Have the Meditation You Are Having.

Track 7. Inquiry: Making A-Statements

Track 8. Contemplation: G-Statements

Track 9. Inquiry: Personal Inquiry

Track 10. Inquiry: Advanced Personal Inquiry

Track 11. Inquiry: The Marvellous Technique of Proxying

Track 12. Inquiry: Who Has Entered My Inner Space?

Track 13. Inquiry: Looking for the Upward Shift Inside

Track 14. Contemplation: Speaking to Your Mind

Track 15. Appendix D: Self-Inquiry for the Four Areas of Life

SELECTED NOTES

OPENING EPIGRAPHS

'They in whom ...': Venkatesananda, trans. *The Supreme Yoga: Yoga Vasiṣṭha* (YV), p. 29.

'... though truth and ...': Donne, 'Satire III' in Abrams, ed. *The Norton Anthology of English Literature*, vol. I, pp. 905–6.

'Good judgment comes ...': Will Rogers, (personal notes).

'Seek what is ...': Maharshi, *Talks with Sri Ramana Maharshi* (TS), p. 12.

LECTURE 1: PERSONAL INQUIRY, PP. 35–59

P. 35   'All paths end ...': Maharshi, (personal notes).

P. 35   'You are so ...': Maharaj, *I Am That, Talks with Sri Nisargadatta Maharaj* (IA), p. 308.

P. 48   '[The esoteric five ...': Kshemaraja in Singh, trans. *Pratyabhijñāhṛdayam* (P), Sutra 11.

P. 48   'When we withdraw ...': P, p. 77.

P. 50   'If a yogi ...': P, pp. 77–8.

LECTURE 2: BE AWARE NOW, PP. 60–84

P. 60   'Inquiry (*vichara*) is ...': TS, p. 27.

P. 60   'Inquiry (the second ...': YV, p. 29.

P. 65   'The primeval one ...': *Katha Upanishad*, I.ii.12, (personal notes).

P. 65   'Little by little ...': *Bhagavad Gita* (BG), VI:25, (personal notes).

P. 66   'It is true ...': YV, p. 336.

P. 66   'Inquiry is the ...': Abhinavagupta, *Tantraloka* (T), Chapter 4, Verse 15, (personal notes).

P. 66   'wish-fulfilling cow which ...': Abhinavagupta, T, (personal notes).

P. 66   'finely sharpened axe ...': ibid.

P. 68   'Therefore, making the ...': Maharshi, (personal notes).

P. 70   'a kind of ...': ibid.

P. 70   'To whom does ...': ibid.

P. 71   'Whatever thoughts arise ...': ibid.

P. 72   'Let whatever strange ...': ibid.

P. 72   'The best discipline ...': ibid.

P. 73   'even though thoughts ...': Utpaladeva,
         *Īśvarapratyabhijñā-Vimarśinī of Abhinavagupta, Doctrine of
         Divine Recognition,* vol. III, Chapter 15, Verse 12.

P. 73   'The eye of ...': YV, p. 29.

P. 76   'Jnanadhishthanam matrika: 'The ...': Singh, trans. *Śiva
         Sūtras* (SS), I.4.

LECTURE 3: THE INNER WORLD, PP. 85–123

P. 85   'Life and all ...': Maharshi, (personal notes).

P. 85   'Bring your Self ...': IA, p. 4.

P. 85   'There in he ...': Abhinavagupta, *Essence of the Exact
         Reality or Paramārthasāra of Abhinavagupta* (EE), Verse 75.

P. 86   'Make the mind ...': Maharshi, (personal notes).

P. 91   'Here, O monks ...': Gautama, the Buddha,
         Mahasatipatthana Suttam, (personal notes).

P. 91   'I have had ...': William Carlos Williams, 'Thursday',
         (personal notes).

P. 94   'Na shivam vidyate ...': *Svacchanda Tantra,* (personal notes).

P. 100   'Aham Brahmasmi: 'I ...': *Brhadaranyaka Upanishad,* 1.4.10,
         in *Yajur Veda, Mahanarayana Upanishad,* (personal notes).

P. 100   'Tat tvam asi: ...': *Chandogya Upanishad* 6.8.7, in *Sama
         Veda, Kaivalya Upanishad,* (personal notes).

LECTURE 4: GROUP-INQUIRY I, PP. 127–171

P. 127   'Inquire into the ...': YV, p. 88.

P. 127   'A friend's eye ...': (personal notes).

P. 129   'O Rama, if ...': YV, p. 27.

P. 138   'What's the point ...': Swami Muktananda, (personal notes).

P. 141   'When the mind ...': Patanjali in Feurstein, trans. *The
         Yoga-Sūtra of Patanjali* (YS), II.33.

P. 143   'Yoga is skill ...': BG, Chapter 3, (personal notes).

P. 168   '*Chaitanyamatma*: 'You are ...': SS, I.1.

LECTURE 5: GROUP-INQUIRY II, PP. 172–216

P. 172   'Rama, such is ...': YV, p. 122.

P. 172   'The state of ...': EE, Verse 60.

P. 172   'The yogi [of ...': Dyczkowski, *The Doctrine of Vibration, An Analysis of the Doctrines and Practices of Kashmir Shaivism*, p. 164.

P. 173   'Silence is ever-speaking ...': TS, p. 210.

P. 175   '*Sharire samharaha kalamam* ...': SS, III.4.

P. 175   '*Te pratiprasava-heyaha sukshmaha* ...': YS, II.10.

P. 176   'An aspirant, enlightened ...': EE, Verse 68.

P. 182   'Om *Purnamadah purnamidam* ...': *The Nectar of Chanting* (NC), p. 68.

P. 196   'Sit in the ...': YS, II.47.

P. 205   '*Bijavadhanam*: 'Focus on ...': SS, III.15.

LECTURE 6: INNER POWER, PP. 219–238

P. 219   'This, indeed, is ...': NC, Verse 97.

P. 219   'Everything is possible ...': Anandamayi Ma, (personal notes).

P. 220   'Thinking sad thoughts ...': *New Idea*, (personal notes).

P. 221   '*Glanir vilunthika dehe* ...': Singh, trans. *Spanda Kārikās* (SK), III.8.

P. 225   '*Aham sukhi cha* ...': SK, I.4.

P. 230   'Oh *sadhus*, oh ...': Kabir, (personal notes).

P. 233   '*Shabdarashi-samutthasya shaktivargasya bhogyatam* ...': SK, I.13.

P. 233   '*Svarupavarane chasya shaktayaha* ...': SK, III.15.

P. 233   '*Seyam kriyatmika shaktihi* ...': SK, III.16.

P. 235   '*Ataha satatam udyuktaha* ...': SK, I.21.

P. 236   '*Tada tasmin mahavyomni* ...': SK, I.25.

SELECTED BIBLIOGRAPHY

Abrams, M. H, general ed. *The Norton Anthology of English Literature.* New York: W. W Norton & Company Inc, 1968.

Dyczkowski, Mark S. G. *The Doctrine of Vibration, An Analysis of the Doctrines and Practices of Kashmir Shaivism.* New York: SUNY, 1987.

Feuerstein, Georg, trans. *The Yoga-Sūtra of Patanjali: A New Translation and Commentary.* Kent: Dawson, 1979.

Maharshi, Ramana. *Talks with Sri Ramana Maharshi.* Tamil Nadu: Sri Ramanasramam, 2003.

Nisargadatta, Maharaj. *I Am That, Talks with Sri Nisargadatta Maharaj.* North Carolina: Acorn Press, 2005.

Pandey, K. C, trans. *Īśvarapratyabhijñā-Vimarśinī of Abhinavagupta, Doctrine of Recognition,* vol. III. Delhi: Motilal Banarsidass, 1986.

Pandit, B. N, trans. *Essence of the Exact Reality or Paramārthasāra of Abhinavagupta.* New Delhi: Munshiram Manoharlal, 1991.

Singh, Jaideva, trans. *Pratyabhijñāhṛdayam, The Secret of Self-Recognition.* Delhi: Motilal Banarsidass, 1977.

_____ , *Śiva Sūtras, The Yoga of Supreme Identity.* Delhi: Motilal Banarsidass, 1979.

_____ , *Spanda Kārikās, The Divine Creative Pulsation.* Delhi: Motilal Banarsidass, 1980.

_____ , *Vijñānabhairava or Divine Consciousness.* Delhi: Motilal Banarsidass, 1979.

Venkatesananda, Swami, trans. *The Supreme Yoga: Yoga Vasiṣṭha.* Himalayas: The Divine Life Society, 1991.

(Author/editor not provided). *The Nectar of Chanting.* Ganeshpuri, India: Gurudev Siddha Peeth, 1980.

GLOSSARY

A-Statement. Accurate statement of present feeling, such as 'I feel happy' or 'I feel sad'. A stage of personal and group-inquiry.

Abhyasa. Positive spiritual effort or practice described by Patanjali. (See also *vairagya*).

Ahimsa. Compassion, kindness.

Alamgrasa. (*lit.* full swallowing) Yogic practice meaning the full swallowing of the world of differentiation and all karmic residue.

Anava mala. Limiting impurity or contraction of will.

Anavopaya. (*lit.* the means of the individual) Yogic action such as service, hatha yoga, *pranayama* and other techniques.

Anitya. Impermanence.

Arati. A ritual during which a flame is waved in front of an image of God. Also the name of the Hindu devotional song which accompanies the ritual.

Asana. (*lit.* posture) Being established in the Self.

Atma vichara. (*lit. atma* = soul; *vichara* = inquiry) Self-inquiry as a means to move towards Self-realisation, most commonly associated with Sri Ramana Maharshi.

Atma vyapti. Turning within to experience the Self. (See also *Shiva vyapti*.)

Avis Process. Questions or statements to point others towards their present experience.

B-Statement. Beneficial statements designed to uplift and positively shift one's present state of being, such as 'I am content' or 'I can do what I need to do easily'. A stage of personal and group-inquiry. G- and D-Statements function as a subset of B-Statements.

Bhakta. (*lit.* devotee, devoted) A lover of God.

Bhakti. (*lit.* devotion) Love of God. Path of devotion.

Big Game, The. A form of Shiva Process to deal with a crisis or recurring block in which the player leaves the room during the process.

Bija. (*lit.* seed) Root cause of the universe, a primary mantra; also the vowels.

Bodhisattva vow. (*lit. bodhi* = enlightened) A Mahayana Buddhist precept seeking enlightenment for all beings.

Brahma. Hindu god of creation and one of trinity including Vishnu and Shiva.

Brahman. Vedantic term for divine Consciousness.

Brahmi. The presiding deity of a group of letters.

Brahmin. High caste in India who take the Vedas as their inspiration and whose daily life is suffused with ritual.

Chakra. (*lit.* wheel) An energy centre of the subtle body.

Chief fault. Gurdjieff's chief feature refers to a central issue around which the false personality revolves.

Consciousness. The supremely independent divine awareness that creates, pervades and supports everything in the cosmos.

D-Statement. 'Doing statements' or homework. A stage of personal and group-inquiry. D- and G-Statements function as a subset of B-Statements.

Dharana. (*lit.* holding) A short meditative exercise.

Divine Shiva Process. A type of Shiva Process in which story is eliminated and the feeling is treated as an entity in itself; a technique related to *shambhavopaya*.

Downward shift. A negative movement of thought and feeling.

Dumping. Indiscriminately spreading a negative feeling accrued in one circumstance.

Dvesha. Aversion.

External considering. Considering the point of view, understanding or emotional state of another person. (See also internal considering.)

False 'I'. The multiple I's of the ordinary self, made up of a false personality, are contrasted by Gurdjieff with the fundamental Self which is consistent and ruled from within by Consciousness.

Feedback. A technique in which A-, B-, G- and D-Statements are given, reflecting the player's present condition and providing upliftment.

First Education. Conventional education of the intellect and personality. (See also Second Education.)

First force. Initiating force, desire, creative impulse. Comprises the first of Gurdjieff's Law of Three. (See also second force and third force.)

Five processes. Five sets of processes comprising creation, sustainment, destruction, concealment and grace at the esoteric, universal and personal levels.

G-Statement. A 'great statement', scriptural statement, God statement or Guru statement. A stage of personal and group-inquiry. G-and D-Statements function as a subset of B-Statements.

Ghee. Clarified butter.

Grasa. (*lit.* swallowing) Consuming.

Group-inquiry. The form of inquiry practised in Shiva Process groups in which feeback features.

Guna. One of three constituents of the material universe. (See also *rajas* and *tamas*.)

Guru. (*lit. gu* = darkness, *ru* = light) A teacher, a Self-realised spiritual master.

Hathapaka. (*lit.* violent digestion) Yogic practice in which reality is devoured whole, in one gulp.

Hathapaka-prasama. Swift and energetic bringing to sameness.

Iccha. The power of will.

Intensive. Meditation workshop in which the Guru bestows divine awakening of the *kundalini* energy. (See also *shaktipat*.)

Internal considering. The negative tendency to see ourselves through others' eyes. (See also external considering.)

Japa. (*lit.* muttering) Constant repetition of the mantra.

Jiva. (*lit.* living being) The individual soul.

Jnana. (*lit.* knowledge) Wisdom or knowledge.

Jnana yoga. Path of discriminating knowledge or wisdom.

Jnani. One who follows the path of discrimination.

Kalaa. Limited ability to do things.

Karma. (*lit.* action) Cause and effect, the rewards or consequences of every thought and action, in this life or in a future life.

Kashmir Shaivism. A philosophy that recognises the entire universe as a manifestation of one Consciousness.

Kriya. (*lit.* movement) The power of action.

Kula-chakra. A group ritual to increase the experience of Consciousness.

Kundalini. (*lit.* coiled one) The inner divine power.

Kundalini shakti. Power of consciousness coiled in latent form in the base of the spine.

Layabhavana. (*lit. laya* = dissolution, *bhava* = attitude) The technique, or attitude, in which gross elements, contractions or energies are dissolved into their underlying, more subtle and higher forms.

Lila. (*lit.* play) The divine sport of Consciousness.

Lord Ganesh. In Hindu mythology, the elephant-headed god who symbolises the removal of obstacles.

Mahavakyas. A collection of 'great statements' selected by Shankaracharya from the Vedas.

Mala. String of beads used when repeating the mantra.

Mantra. (*lit. manana* = mind, *tranam* = that which protects) Sacred word or phrase invested with the power to transform the person who repeats it.

Matrika. (*lit.* unknown mother) Letters and sounds, the inherent power of letters and words that give rise to language and knowledge.

Neelakantha. (*lit.* Blue-throated One) A name for Shiva. The one whose throat turned blue from swallowing the poison that contaminated the ocean.

Neti, neti. (*lit.* not this, not this) A Vedantic attitude of negating the objective universe until only supreme Consciousness remains.

Nirbija samadhi. (lit. *nirbija* =seed; lit. *samadhi* = meditative absorption) An experience of deep meditation free of thought constructs. (See also *nirvikalpa samadhi.*)

Nirvikalpa. (*lit.* no thought-constructs) The state of mind that is free of thoughts.

Nirvikalpa samadhi. A deep experience of meditation in which the mind is free of thoughts.

Peculiar. A person whose primary tendency is emotional in the typology of Solid-Vital-Peculiar.

Personal inquiry. The form of inquiry practised within yourself during meditation.

Prakasha. (*lit.* light) The light of supreme Consciousness.

Prana. The vital breath or energy, life force.

Pranayama. Yogic breathing.

Proxying. A Shiva Process technique for identifying and positively influencing another person's emotional state.

Puja. (*lit.* worship) Ritual worship of God.

Raga. Attachment, desire and a sense of lack.

Raja yoga. (lit. raja = royal; yoga = union) A type of yoga concerned mainly with cultivating the mind using meditation.

Rajas. One of the three *gunas*, the principle of activity and passion. (See also *tamas.*)

Rama. (lit. darkness) Legendary king of ancient India, considered in Hinduism to be the seventh avatar of India.

Right speech. (lit. right = coherence, ideal) One of the Ways of the Buddha's noble eightfold path, comprising right view, right intention, right speech, right action, right livelihood, right effort, right mindfulness, right concentration. A practical guide said to lead to the end of suffering. The eightfold path forms the fourth part of the four noble truths.

Sadhana. Spiritual practice; the yogic process of transformation.

Sadhu. (*lit.* good one) Holy one.

Sahaja samadhi. The natural state of a Self-realised being living in harmony with the Self or God.

Sahasrara. The energy centre at the crown of the head.

Samadhi. Highest level of meditative attainment where the mind becomes merged with divine Consciousness.

Samkhya. A system of philosophy that recognises two realities; matter and Consciousness.

Samsara. Transmigratory existence, the world process.

Samsarin. A transmigratory being.

Samskara. Impressions.

Satchitananda. (*lit. sat* = being, existence, *chit* = Consciousness, *ananda* = bliss) Ultimate Consciousness that underlies all as the absolute state of existence, dwelling in bliss.

Satsang. (*lit. sat* = truth, *sanga* = company) Gathering in the name of a great being or principle. Spending time with a realised being or a spiritually minded group or community.

Satya. Truth.

Second Education. Internal, or spiritual/psychological education. (See also First Education.)

Second force. Difficulty, resistance, blocks or tension. Comprises the second of Gurdjieff's Law of Three. (See also first force and third force.)

Self. The divine conscious essence of a person. Underlying Consciousness that is everywhere.

Self-inquiry. A method of meditation using inner questioning, as practised in personal inquiry, private sessions and group-inquiry.

Self-realisation. The goal of *sadhana*. Being permanently established in the state of connection with the inner Self.

Self-remembering. A term coined by Gurdjieff meaning an act of awareness to remember the higher Self which is ever-present but subsumed by the false personality. (See also false 'I', chief fault.)

Shaivite. A follower of Shiva; practitioner of Kashmir Shaivism.

Shakti. The divine energy that creates, maintains and dissolves the universe. Also, spiritual energy, the female or dynamic aspect of Consciousness.

Shakti Process. A therapeutic form of Shiva Process which focuses on personal, unconscious or conscious hurts and is especially suited to people suffering from addictions, negative thinking or blocks.

Shaktipat. (*lit.* descent of grace) Initiation or spiritual awakening of the kundalini energy by the Guru.

Shaktopaya. (*lit.* the means of Shakti) Using the highest thought and language such as mantra or prayer to sort out concepts, understandings and emotions. (See also *upaya.*)

Shambhavopaya. (*lit.* the means of Shiva) Using pure will to stay in the thought-free state of pure Consciousness. (See also *upaya.*)

Shanti-prasama. A gradual and peaceful bringing to oneness.

Shifting statement. A-, B-, G- and D-Statements that cause a significant shift.

Shiva. Hindu god of destruction and one of trinity including Brahma and Vishnu. Also refers to divine Consciousness.

Shiva Process. A method of personal and group-inquiry designed to unblock tensions and move the seeker into a higher, more peaceful state.

Shiva vyapti. Experiencing the Divine in the world. (See also *atma vyapti.*)

Siddha. One who has the highest attainment, perfected being.

Solid. A person whose primary tendency is intellectual in the typology of Solid-Vital-Peculiar.

Spanda principle. The principle of the expansive vibration, or upward shift, of Consciousness.

Sutra. A short aphoristic statement.

Tamas. One of the three *gunas*, the principle of dullness and sloth. (See also *rajas.*)

Tantra. A spiritual technique that finds divinity in the world; often contrasted to Vedic or Vedantic.

Tao. (*lit.* path or way) Living in the Tao refers to living in alignment with the natural order of the universe.

Tapasya. (*lit.* to heat or burn) Spiritual practices of austerity and discipline.

Tattva. In Shaivite cosmology, one of 36 levels of creation or Consciousness.

Tearing thought. A negative or limiting statement.

Third force. Grace or the power that removes a block or resistance. Comprises the third of Gurdjieff's Law of Three. (See also first force and second force).

Tonglen. (*lit.* taking and giving) A Tibetan Buddhist meditation practice in which the practitioner visualises taking on the suffering of others, and giving to others their own happiness.

Turiya. (*lit.* fourth) The fourth state of Consciousness, beyond waking, dream and deep sleep.

Unmesha. (*lit.* unfoldment) Revelation of the essential nature of the Divine, the expansive upward shift of feeling when the Self is contacted.

Upanishad. Spiritual contemplations of the Vedas, forming the core spiritual thought of Vedantic Hinduism (See also Vedas).

Upaya. Spiritual or yogic method, means or path by which the individual soul returns to pure Consciousness.

Upward shift. A positive movement of thought and feeling.

Vairagya. (*lit.* aversion) Yogic dispassion or letting go; asceticism. Negative spiritual effort or practice described by Patanjali (See also *abhyasa*).

Vedanta. Spiritual philosophy that says Consciousness

underlies the universe, and the world is an illusion.

Vedas. (*lit.* to know) Corpus of Sanskrit texts, the oldest sacred texts of Hinduism, said to be directly revealed from God.

Vikalpa. Thought-form, conceptualisation.

Vimarsha. The eternal Self-awareness of divine Consciousness.

Viparyaya. One of the sections of the *vrittis*, or forms of thought, meaning misapprehension.

Vishnu. Hindu god of sustainment and one of trinity including Brahma and Shiva.

Vital. A person whose primary tendency is activity in the typology of Solid-Vital-Peculiar.

Viveka. Yogic discrimination.

Witness-consciousness. A meditative practice in which the mind is observed from a distance.

Wrong crystallisation. Gurdjieff's term to describe when spiritual growth on the basis of false personality increases ego rather than eliminates it.

Yagna. (*lit. yag* = to sacrifice) Ancient Vedic fire ritual.

Yamas. Disciplines; self-control.

Yantra. (*lit.* support or restrain) A mystical diagram used as a centring device or as a symbolic representation of the deity.

Yoga. (*lit.* union) Spiritual practice, the path of spirituality.

Yogi. One who practises yoga; a seeker.

Zen. A school of Mahayana Buddhism that emphasises practice and experiential wisdom.

INDEX

ABOUT SWAMI SHANKARANANDA

SWAMI SHANKARANANDA (SWAMIJI) is a Self-realised meditation master who has taught thousands of people to meditate. He grew up in Brooklyn, New York, and as a graduate of both Columbia and New York Universities, he began a promising career in English Literature at Indiana University. In the late '60s, a dramatic turn of events profoundly altered the direction of his life and led him to India in search of the great sages.

Swamiji spent time with the mysterious Neem Karoli Baba, the wisdom-teacher Sri Nisargadatta Maharaj, and the holy mother Anandamayi Ma. He practised Buddhist Vipassana meditation with Sri Goenka and hatha and raja yoga with Baba Hari Dass. His search ended in 1971 when he met the powerful and charismatic Swami Muktananda (Baba), a renowned master of yoga and meditation, under whom he studied for 12 years. In 1977, Swamiji was initiated into the monastic Saraswati teaching order of swamis. In 1991, he founded the Shiva School of Meditation and Yoga, near Melbourne, Australia, where he currently resides. In 2007, Swamiji was inaugurated in India as a Mahant (spiritual leader) in the Pancha Agni Akhada, one of the six Akhadas of the ancient ascetic sects of Shaivism, in recognition of his spiritual attainment.

As one of the world's foremost teachers of Kashmir Shaivism, he has integrated this powerful philosophy into Western culture. His highly acclaimed book, *Consciousness Is Everything: The Yoga of Kashmir Shaivism*, presents the wisdom of this tradition in a form that helps readers investigate and deepen their own Consciousness. He is also the author of the Australian bestseller *Happy for No Good Reason*, a comprehensive manual of meditation and guidebook for everyday life, and *Carrot in My Ear*, a compilation of questions and answers about spiritual practice and philosophy. Other titles by Swamiji include a five-CD lecture series, *The Yoga of Gurdjieff*, and the audio and video series, *Great Beings*.

Swamiji says that Self-realisation, upliftment, wisdom and love are available here and now, in this moment. To integrate yoga and spirituality into worldly life, he developed the Shiva Process Self-inquiry as a practical method to improve relationships, increase understanding and achieve personal freedom. His reputation as a master draws national and international recognition as students from around the world are inspired by his profound teachings and compassionate and wise guidance.